"The stronger your immune function is, the better equipped your body is to fight infection and disease."

— Dr. Grace McComsey and
Dr. Andrew Myers

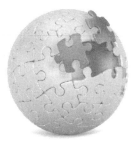

SIMPLIFYING
the
COVID PUZZLE

How Two Essential Vitamins
***Fortify** the Immune System*

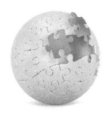

DR. GRACE McCOMSEY
AND
DR. ANDREW MYERS

Ballast Books, LLC
Washington, D.C.
BallastBooks.com

Simplifying the COVID Puzzle
How Two Essential Vitamins Fortify the Immune System
Copyright © 2021 by Health Value Communications

ISBN: 978-1-955026-00-0
Library of Congress Control Number has been applied for.

Cover Design: Mirko Pohle
Interior Design: Fusion Creative Works, FusionCW.com
Book Production: Aloha Publishing LLC, AlohaPublishing.com

Published by Ballast Books, LLC

For more information, bulk orders, appearances, or speaking requests, please email info@ballastbooks.com

Printed in Canada

Dedication

With the hope that we can reestablish our trust in science and the objective of bringing proactive, preventive care to people everywhere.

Contents

The Immune Response to COVID-19
Nutritional Deficiency Affects the Immune Response
How Nutritional Deficiency Affects the COVID-19
    Immune Response

The Well-Known Benefits of Vitamin D
The Emerging Data on Vitamin D and COVID-19

The Recognized Benefits of Vitamin K2
Vitamin K2's Effect on Inflammation
The Emerging Data on Vitamin K and COVID-19
The First Link Between Vitamin K and COVID-19
Vitamin K2 MK-7

The Need for Vitamin K2 With Vitamin D
Building Stronger Immunity Through Better Nutrition
The Prevalence of Vitamin D and Vitamin K2 Deficiencies
Getting Enough of Vitamins D and K2
Our Recommendation: Supplement to Reach Sufficient
    Levels of Vitamins D and K2
Vitamin K2 MK-7 Supplement Standards and Purity

Other Essential Nutrients to Boost Your Health
Five Daily Habits to Strengthen Your Immune System

Foreword

The ability to keep your body well and help it heal are priorities for anyone who wants to take charge of their health, especially in times of widespread disease. While government and health department guidelines help, there is a missing ingredient in the recipe for preventing and healing from viral infections: **building a healthy immune system**. *Simplifying the COVID Puzzle: How Two Essential Vitamins Fortify the Immune System* gives you the tools to strengthen your immune system.

Preventive medicine and healing science are "inside jobs." You have an immune system army (ISA) made up of trillions of cells. If your ISA could shout—it does, but we don't tend to listen—your army would say, "Feed us well and train us well and we'll fight better for you." Dr. McComsey's and Dr. Myers' book explains why feeding and caring for your body well should be a priority for everyone.

I'm a show-me-the-science type of doctor. I won't prescribe any pill or teach any skill that isn't supported by science. In this book, Dr. McComsey, a university professor of infectious diseases and a clinical researcher, and Dr. Myers, a naturopathic physician with globally recognized expertise, combine their decades of experience. They explain the important and recently discovered science behind their message—that we need to focus more on our immune system health by supplying our bodies with the required micronutrients we may not get from our diets.

You will learn how to equip your immune system to confront infectious diseases and other immune system challenges that you encounter every day. These doctors have spent their professional careers studying the immune system. As you utilize the strategies they share, it will be as if you're saying at the cellular level, "No access granted!" to viruses and invaders.

This book is a unique blend of science and common sense. The two star nutrients it focuses on are vitamin D and vitamin K2, partners in immune system health. Unfortunately, many of us don't get enough of these two nutrients to build our immune systems. I especially loved learning how the roles of these two nutrients combine to provide greater benefits than they can alone, creating *synergy*—an important scientific principle that means they work better together.

One of my favorite teachings is how to have better blood vessel health. Every organ of your body is only as healthy as the blood flow to it. Vitamins D and K2 keep blood flow less sticky and the arteries more flexible. Better blood flow equals healthier tissues.

Read it, do it, and feel it—you'll be glad you did.

— **William Sears, M.D.**

Founder of AskDrSears.com and author of *The Healthy Brain Book: An All-Ages Guide to a Calmer, Happier, Sharper You*

Preface

As I write this book, we are in a new world—one remade by a pandemic that has reprioritized and upended the way we live. As COVID-19 has swept across the globe, it has brought new dangers, new fears, and a new reality with it. My life has certainly changed, and I would venture to say yours has, too.

I've spent decades working as a clinical research physician specializing in infectious disease. I currently lead the Clinical Research Center for the University Hospitals (U.H.) Health System in Cleveland, Ohio, a network of 18 hospitals that serves over 1.5 million patients. I am also a Professor of Pediatrics and Medicine at Case Western Reserve University, Cleveland, Ohio. Teaching and mentoring students and young doctors have always been my passion, along with research.

As soon as news broke of the severe acute respiratory syndrome coronavirus 2 (SARS-CoV-2) and resulting COVID-19 disease, my research team began preparing.

Research is ongoing and we currently have over 200 studies related to COVID-19 underway. While more research is needed, we have uncovered some useful guidelines for treatment of the disease, including some fascinating details about vitamin D and vitamin K2.

The interactions of vitamins D and K2 with the immune system are the primary focus of this book. It is remarkable that little attention, even among doctors, has been given to the potential of vitamin K2 and I am committed to changing that.

In 2020, my research team started a correlational study around vitamins D and K2 in COVID-19 patients. We specifically wanted to assess whether having optimal vitamin D and vitamin K2 status prior to or at the time someone gets COVID-19 would lessen their risk of severe disease.

The amazing results of this correlational research further propelled our interest in writing this book.

My background is in adult and pediatric infectious disease with an emphasis in human immunodeficiency virus (HIV), which means I've spent much of my life investigating viruses and the body's immune response. Dr. Andrew Myers is a naturopathic physician who has concentrated much of his life's work on nutrition. I have always been fascinated with healthy nutrition and nutritional supplements as a way to support and optimize the immune system. As we learn more about COVID and how different individuals respond to the virus, Dr. Myers and I see the potential for our paths to come together to inform a smart approach.

Nothing offered here is a magic solution. Plenty of unanswered questions around COVID remain. Research needs to continue, and scientists around the world, including myself and my team, are committed to learning as much as possible. Despite all that is left to learn, there are tangible things we can do to strengthen our immune systems that will likely keep us safer during this pandemic and flu season, and even into the next pandemic. We're incredibly excited to share some of those things with you. Now. Because now is when this conversation needs to get started.

Dr. Myers and I hope you find this information valuable and let it empower you to make decisions that keep you and your family as healthy as possible.

Introduction

You probably picked up this book because you're worried about yourself or a loved one getting sick. In the middle of a serious global pandemic, this is an understandable concern. So I don't want to hold you in any suspense—I want you to know, immediately and directly, what has potential to help you and your family right now.

This is what I can tell you.

Research is showing us that we can better understand the COVID puzzle by bringing our attention to two key micronutrients that many people are deficient in and which are essential for strong immune function. These micronutrients are especially important for the body to deal with viruses like SARS-CoV-2, the culprit virus in COVID-19 infection. These two micronutrients are vitamin D and vitamin K2. Each of these is a critical piece of this puzzle on its own as well as in synergistic combination with the other.

While some people love the idea of supplementing with vitamins, some tend to dismiss them. The reality is that vitamins can be incredibly powerful and they deserve our attention.

We are learning that vitamins D and K2 are essential to the immune system. To be clear, they do not cure COVID-19. What we're learning points to their power in disease prevention and helping the immune system function at its best. When the immune system is provided with adequate vitamins D and K2, it has a better chance of fighting off the disease before a severe outcome develops. Dr. Myers and I see this preventative power as reason for celebration—and action. We believe that widespread supplementation with vitamin D and vitamin K2 should be part of our pandemic response strategy, along with masks, social distancing, and vaccine and treatment development.

Emerging knowledge around vitamins D and K2 is giving us a chance to save lives, keep more people out of hospitals, and help people strengthen their general immunity, all with something widely available, inexpensive, and safe.

We wrote this book to help you navigate this particular moment, a time when our lives are being changed by the pandemic, but the book is about more than just COVID-19. Vitamins D and K2 are so needed in this crisis because they support the body's immune system. They provide it with the resources it needs to operate at its peak. That's what the book is about—how to strengthen your immunity through a better understanding of the importance of nutrition and healthy lifestyle choices.

Our recommendations are simple, but it's important to share the significant research and context behind them. The following chapters will cover this in greater detail, because the more you understand the larger story of immunity and nutrition around vitamins D and K2, the more equipped you'll be to make the best choices for your health.

We'll start by taking a moment to set the context. I'll share some of my story and how we got to this point in our study of vitamins D and K2. Next, we'll move into nutrition and how you can use nutrients and lifestyle to build a foundation for strong immunity. Then we'll dive into the immune system itself. We'll look at the roles vitamins D and K2 play along the way. From there, we'll get into the bulk of the research around the emerging puzzle pieces that show why vitamin D and vitamin K2 are so important right now. We'll look at how common deficiency is and how to get enough of these essential nutrients. Then we'll round things out with suggestions on how to bring all of this together in a holistic way to build strong immunity.

From there, it's up to you.

CHAPTER 1

Piecing Together the COVID-19 Puzzle

Since the COVID-19 pandemic began, I have worked to answer the question "What simple, logical things can we do right now to help?"

While much is left to be done, enough information has been gathered to say with confidence that we all have the power to make a difference for ourselves. By deliberately choosing what we do to care for ourselves every day, we can strengthen our immune systems to protect us from infectious diseases.

This may sound simple, but we have evidence to back it up: live a healthier lifestyle and ensure you get the nutrients you need, with an emphasis on obtaining optimum levels of vitamin D and vitamin K2.

These two vitamins are essential missing pieces for both the COVID-19 and the immunity puzzles. This key takeaway has a lot of science behind that simplicity, though, and the more you know, the better equipped you'll be to make the best decisions for yourself.

As an infectious diseases physician, I heard from colleagues for years that a pandemic was definitely in our future. Expectations were for a bad flu—but the virulence of COVID-19 surprised many of us. We must navigate this situation with the understanding that there will be more pandemics in the future, and we need to prepare for the next one.

 COVID-19 is definitely not the last pandemic the world will face.

Understanding better the roles of vitamins D and K2 can help us weather the current situation and the next pandemic, whatever it may be.

In the introduction, we dropped right into the high points and now I want to step back to explore the layers of science and the story behind them. Unfolding these layers will help you understand why our recommendations are so important.

I'll start with a small piece of what led me to my work as a doctor and to write this book. In my years as a physician, I've learned that relationship and context are important, so I want you to understand the context from which this research emerged.

My Path to Working With Infectious Diseases

Today, I work primarily with HIV patients, some of whom I've known for decades. They trust me to guide them as they navigate difficult situations, in part because we've taken a journey together. We've built a relationship over time based on the human stuff—real presence and connection and listening—as much as the essential medical care. They respect my judgement and know that I really care about them. Because I do.

Making a difference in my patients' lives is an important and meaningful part of my work—but it's not the only part. I went into research because I love doing all I can to help as many people as I can. Writing this book is one way of doing that, to help you learn more about how your body works so you can make choices that contribute to your health and well-being.

All of this is information I would extend to my patients, family, and friends, who I believe would value it in part because they know me and feel my care for them. I can't know each of you reading this book, but you matter to me, too. While we can't build the same kind of relationship that I do with my clinic patients, we will take a short journey together as we share this information. It's helpful and important to ground that journey in the human stuff—the why—so I'd like to start by sharing some of my own story with you.

I grew up in Lebanon during a civil war, which meant that much of life and human interaction around me was defined by what side you were on. But not everyone appeared to see the world this way. My parents didn't, and neither did those in medicine. I saw from a young age that medicine seemed to be a way to help people regardless of what faction they came from, and this made a deep, lasting impression on me.

I didn't know I wanted to be a doctor right away. With a real love for math and physics, I initially felt called to be an engineer. My parents encouraged me to think about medicine, though, and after I started volunteering with the Red Cross in high school, I began to seriously consider it.

In Lebanon, you commit to a university path around age 17. After doing well on the tests for both engineering and medical school, I still didn't know what I wanted to do. It was a tough decision but ultimately the sense of wanting to help people, all people, like I'd seen doctors and nurses do during the war, tipped me into embarking on the path to medicine. I became enamored with it.

The first few years of med school were interesting. I'd studied very little biology in high school so it was mostly new for me, and I like learning new things. The real moment when I knew I'd chosen the right path, though, was when we started the clinical side. Once I started to see patients, I had no doubt this was what I wanted to do with my life.

I planned to go to Paris for my residency after I graduated, because in the French Lebanese school system I was a part of, that was the expected next step. I was even signed up to work in a hospital there. Then during one of my last rotations, I was placed with a Lebanese physician who had trained in New Jersey and was American board certified in infectious disease. I was fascinated by his thinking. He utilized a simpler, more logical approach to solving patients' problems, one that worked just as well or better than the more complicated French approach I was used to. Seeing this really affected me, and I started to wonder if I should go to the U.S. to finish my own training.

My parents thought I was crazy, and I didn't blame them. To begin with, I didn't speak a word of English. On top of that, at the time it was nearly impossible for a Lebanese citizen to get a U.S. visa. But the U.S.-trained physician I encountered during my final rotations had made such an impression on me that I decided I wanted to see if I could do it anyway.

Since the U.S. embassy in Lebanon was closed due to the war, I had to go to the neighboring country of Syria to apply for a visa. When I arrived, the woman there said, "You know we're not giving out visas now, right?" I said yes, I'd heard, but I wanted to try. I candidly explained why I wanted to go. She asked me if I knew anyone there and I told her I didn't, besides an uncle I didn't know well. He'd moved there years before.

She took a moment to take all of this in, along with the apparent fact that I didn't speak any English (made clear by our conversation needing to be held in Arabic). Then she said, "Okay. You're the only one today and the only one from Lebanon in months, but yes." I think she was intrigued by my drive to go.

My parents could hardly believe it. Even after getting the visa, there were still the questions of language and getting a residency slot. I simply said, "I'll go, I'll learn English, and I'll get a slot. I'll just do it."

And that's what I did.

I came to the U.S. and stayed with my uncle in New York, where I learned the language fairly quickly. I was surrounded by his English-speaking friends, and my knowledge of French helped me, too. Within a few months, I got a residency slot in New Jersey, and then after visiting a friend at Case Western Reserve University in Cleveland, I decided to transfer my residency there and specialize in infectious disease. I've been in Cleveland and at Case Western—first as a resident fellow and then as faculty—ever since.

The COVID Puzzle

I share this story in part because what brought me to the U.S. is what still drives my approach to medicine today.

My early interest in mechanical engineering has translated into a deep interest in puzzles. I'm drawn to work with diseases that have no cure and with questions that don't have easy answers.

In infectious disease research and treatment, our work isn't based on procedures. It's a specialty that's not focused on just one organ, so we think a lot about the patient as a whole. Everything is at play, including someone's mental health—it's all connected. I also try to find the unique aspect of everything, even with common problems, because every person has a unique body. As a researcher and a clinician I'm always asking, "What do we not know? And what do I need to do to help answer that question?"

The approach I saw in the U.S.-trained physician I encountered in Lebanon became the way that I, too, practice medicine and think through the puzzles of my work. When I see an opportunity to go from A to B in a straight line, I take it. I do that when I give a presentation explaining my research; I want everyone to understand me and my findings.

There's also an elegance to finding that groove of simplicity within complexity. I believe there's great value in approaching a problem by first considering those simple, logical things we can do to help.

Now here we are with COVID-19.

People everywhere are finding themselves susceptible and sick. In response to the threat, our previous ways of working and connecting have shifted. Kids are often out of school, we work from home when we can, and we share celebrations over Zoom. People have lost their jobs and the economy has been shaken.

Almost everyone I know has been affected by the pandemic on a deep level. We're isolated. Many feel scared and powerless. People are dying.

A friend recently told me her 6-year-old son said he didn't really remember what it was like before the virus. That's a sad thing to hear. It also pains me to think of the elderly, spending what may be their last years alone and in fear.

It's a hard way for all of us to live, and we don't know how long it will last. We also don't know what long-term effects we'll feel individually and as a society.

When the pandemic first came, it reminded me in many ways of the war days of my childhood. There was a feeling of doom in the air. We experienced a shortage of supplies and food. I saw rows and rows of empty shelves, just like I'd seen whenever another round of fighting broke out. On a personal level, it felt scary.

On a professional level, we got to work fast. My research team started preparing in January, as soon as we heard that the virus was in China and spreading; we were the first to start COVID-19 therapeutic studies in the Cleveland area. Within four months, we had 130 COVID-19 studies underway and by December 2020, we had more than 200.

Everyone was working night and day to advance the research, get funding, and do things that could help people. It was intense and stressful, but we all did it because we needed to. With COVID, there were (and are) so many questions, and we had nothing to offer. Research was our only hope. That awareness brought out great things from everyone—medical teams, branches of government, support staff, patients. We were able to do things faster than we ever believed possible, without cutting corners on safety.

Someone outside the medical profession recently told me that because the COVID-19 vaccines had been developed so fast, she questioned if they would be safe. I understand why she might think that. When you see development that frequently takes more than five years, happen—start to finish—in nine months, you might wonder if some important steps were left out. As someone who has been in the thick of things, I told her that ensuring safety and proving efficacy has stayed at the forefront of the process. Nothing there has changed. It's simply been a matter of less red tape and more urgency.

At my hospital center, I saw this firsthand. The typical time it takes to initiate a study was reduced drastically. For example, with our first trial of the Remdesivir antiviral, it took us two and a half days from the time we got the package and paperwork from the sponsor to the time we were ready to start. This process usually takes two to four months. These sorts of shifts have allowed great things to happen.

Research is moving fast, and we're sharing it just as fast, because we need it now.

My research team is currently exploring several questions around the disease. Some of the most exciting research I'm involved in concerns vitamin K2, and our findings have been quite remarkable. We're also looking at vitamin D, zinc, therapeutics, different antibodies, different antivirals (some oral), and preventive studies with monoclonal antibodies. We're examining possible treatments, looking at prevention, and aiming to understand different facets of COVID-19 and what the long-term consequences are.

The long-term consequences are very important as the number of people who have had the disease grows, because having COVID-19 means more than just a few days or weeks of symptoms. More and more, the concern is shifting to what we call "long haulers," people who recover slowly and only partially from COVID.

From the start, this disease has been a puzzle—one that grips my mind as a researcher.

It's a powerful example of how different each body is. Most people recover from COVID-19, but many people still die. It's not even always the elderly or those with obvious and extensive health problems—what we call comorbidities. Seemingly healthy young people can get surprisingly sick. So I ask, what is going on beneath the surface that makes our individual bodies respond so differently to the disease? Is there anything we can do that will help our bodies respond better?

I also wonder what will happen to the millions of people in the world who've had the virus? What, if any, are the long-term effects of the disease? Today, that answer isn't clear, but some incidences are causes for concern. Up to 30 percent of people who recover from COVID-19 continue to have symptoms for months after—we call this long COVID. They may have heart or lung issues, joint pain, or neurocognitive issues including a decline in memory and cognition. Some feel chronic fatigue or chronic muscle aches. Colleagues across the nation have also told me of new-onset diabetes and new-onset hypothyroidism in people who never had those problems but suddenly develop them after they've recovered from COVID-19. There's even a question of whether the virus could affect fertility in men and women.

We don't know what this will all look like years from now because as I write this, the disease was identified just over a year ago. To really understand the long-term effects, we have to keep studying those effects over an extended period of time. As we study the long-term effects, there are serious questions we as researchers need to consider.

The COVID-19 disease creates a state of acute inflammation. Are the aftereffects of the disease the result of lingering systemic inflammation? In my research I use certain inflammation markers to track systemic inflammation. If you recover from COVID, what happens to inflammation markers that used to be 10 or 20 times the acceptable range in the body? Do they really go away? And if they do, how long does that take? Does persisting inflammation from COVID link to any end-organ diseases, like heart or brain disease, that are known to be tied to inflammation in my own research? Many family members of sick COVID patients have commented that their loved one now seems 10 years older. It would not be unprecedented if the inflammation caused by severe COVID could induce premature aging, like we see with the chronic inflammation associated with treated, controlled HIV infection.

What is an end-organ disease?

An end organ can be thought of as a target organ—the organ that is ultimately affected by a process or disease. These are often major organs such as the heart, kidneys, lungs, or liver.

Exploring these questions will help us determine the full extent of the damage from this pandemic and help us better understand the question at the root of all of this: What changes take place in the body of someone who gets COVID-19?

Existing Countermeasures

As we think, research, and continue to move through this pandemic, my mind keeps returning to this question: What simple, logical things can we do to help?

The more we learn and advance, the better we'll be able to answer that question. We can begin to answer it right now too.

What You've Already Heard About: Masks and Social Distancing

First, there's what has already been communicated from official sources: masks and social distancing. We've all heard these recommendations but I must emphasize them because they're important. At times there's been confusion around them. Handwashing has also been mentioned with instructions on how to do it properly, but that has been less controversial.

COVID-19: Preventive Measures
Know how it spreads

COVID-19 spreads easily from person to person, mainly by the following routes:

- Between people who are in close contact with one another (within 6 feet).
- Through respiratory droplets produced when an infected person coughs, sneezes, breathes, sings, or talks.
  - Respiratory droplets cause infection when they are inhaled or deposited on mucous membranes, such as those that line the inside of the nose and mouth.
- People who are infected but do not have symptoms can also spread the virus to others.

Wash your hands often

- Wash your hands often with soap and water for at least 20 seconds especially after you have been in a public place, or after blowing your nose, coughing, or sneezing.
- If soap and water are not readily available, use a hand sanitizer that contains at least 60% alcohol. Cover all surfaces of your hands and rub them together until they feel dry.
- Avoid touching your eyes, nose, and mouth with unwashed hands.

Avoid close contact

- Put six feet of distance between yourself and people who don't live in your household.

Cover your mouth and nose with a mask when around others

- Masks help prevent you from getting or spreading the virus.

Cover coughs and sneezes

- Always cover your mouth and nose with a tissue when you cough or sneeze or use the inside of your elbow and do not spit.

Clean and disinfect

- Clean and disinfect frequently touched surfaces daily.

Monitor your health daily

- Be alert for symptoms.

Don't purposely put yourself at risk

- Medical experts say bars are places with a high risk of easily spreading COVID-19.
  - Among other factors, this is primarily due to the fact that they're spots where large numbers of people gather indoors with little ventilation over long periods of time.
  - When people are drinking in a bar, they can often become too relaxed, leading to safety rules and protocols falling by the wayside.

*https://www.cdc.gov/coronavirus/2019-ncov/prevent-getting-sick/prevention.html

At the start of the pandemic, people were told not to wear masks and sometimes even told that wearing one may be worse than not wearing one at all. One large study showed that masks didn't work, and a lot of people heard about that. The problem was that the study didn't take into account what type of mask was worn, and this makes a real difference. Gaiter masks, for example, don't work well and can sometimes be worse than nothing. Yet other masks, such as N95 masks, work extremely well. Then as the pandemic continued, masks were supposed to be reserved for healthcare workers; if you wore one, you were doing something selfish. After that, as time went on, not wearing one became selfish. The guidance from authorities changed over time and was sometimes confusing.

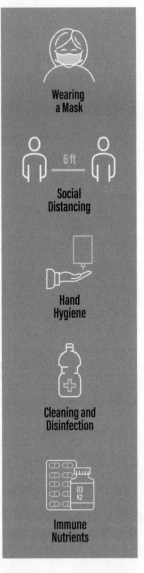

Wearing
a Mask

Social
Distancing

Hand
Hygiene

Cleaning and
Disinfection

Immune
Nutrients

We've also been told to practice social distancing, but there have been cases when authorities have seemed to relax that recommendation or were inconsistent in implementing it.

The story has changed a lot, and frankly, transparency has been lacking around why it's changing. It doesn't help that the pandemic has also become politicized, which has contributed to distrust.

However, this pandemic goes far beyond politics. It doesn't matter to me as a physician what your political loyalties are or where you get your news. I believe you and every person on this planet deserve to know all you can.

The bottom line is that masks can protect us and others 50-70 percent of the time. In my mind, there's no question that's a good thing. The practice of social distancing is probably even more important than masks when it comes to reducing transmission.

We should all be doing these things.

That being said, on their own, these strategies are unlikely to be enough. There's probably no single practice or treatment that can end this pandemic.

CDC Guidelines for COVID-19

COVID-19 affects different people in different ways. Infected people have had a wide range of symptoms reported—from mild symptoms to severe illness. Symptoms may appear **2-14 days after exposure to the virus.** People with these symptoms may have COVID-19:

- Fever or chills
- Cough
- Shortness of breath or difficulty breathing
- Fatigue
- Muscle or body aches
- Headache
- New loss of taste or smell
- Sore throat
- Congestion or runny nose
- Nausea or vomiting
- Diarrhea

Look for emergency warning signs* for COVID-19. If someone is showing any of these signs, seek emergency medical care immediately:

- Trouble breathing
- Persistent pain or pressure in the chest
- New confusion
- Inability to wake or stay awake
- Bluish lips or face

*This list does not include all possible symptoms. Please call your medical provider for any other symptoms that are severe or concerning to you.

These guidelines are current as of February 2021.

https://www.cdc.gov/coronavirus/2019-ncov/symptoms-testing/symptoms.html

Commonsense Guidelines for the COVID-19 Pandemic

At the start of the pandemic, it wasn't always clear what you were supposed to do and for how long, when you had symptoms of any sickness or were exposed to COVID-19. Guidelines have been clarified in most areas, but in case your local guidelines aren't easy to find or interpret, here is a brief summary.

When you feel sick:

When feeling symptoms of any sickness at all (whether it specifically seems to indicate COVID-19 or not), stay home.

If you want to get tested, go in for testing and then quarantine until you get a negative result. If you get a positive result, quarantine for 10 days from the start of your symptoms *and* until any severe symptoms have passed.

If you feel comfortable taking care of yourself at home and don't want to get tested, quarantine for 10 days from the start of your symptoms *and* until any severe symptoms have passed.

Seek medical care if you need it. Get to the hospital immediately whenever you experience one of the emergency warning signs listed in the CDC guidelines, covered in the preceding section.

To be clear, these are not the only symptoms of COVID-19; rather, these are *emergency* symptoms that indicate you need to go to the hospital right away.

When you've been exposed:

Quarantine for 14 days from the time of exposure, whether you develop symptoms or not.

If you develop symptoms, quarantine for 10 days from the start of your symptoms *and* until any severe symptoms have passed.

Emerging Solutions

We Need More Than a Vaccine

Vaccine development is crucial, and it's been amazing to see how quickly it has happened. Yet we need to remember vaccines aren't necessarily an immediate or assured solution. First of all, to see a large effect, we need over 70 percent of the population to have immunity, either from the vaccine or from having had the disease. Typically, the millions of people who've gotten sick and recovered would factor into this percentage, but with COVID-19, we don't know how long their immunity lasts. It's looking like antibodies may sometimes decrease significantly after only three or four months. (However, other parts of the immune system involving T-cells may offer a more lasting immunity.) If we can't rely on the immunity of those who've had COVID, that 70 percent threshold of immunity needs to be reached primarily from the vaccine. That will require an exceptionally high level of acceptance from the public, and we're not there yet.

In addition, the long-term efficacy of the vaccine is unknown. New strains of the virus are also being identified, which we hope the vaccine will also protect against, but we can't say for sure yet. Research is actively happening to inform us. However, even in best-case scenarios, a vaccine almost certainly won't remove all threat of the virus.

I believe the vaccine will be a significant part of our pandemic approach, but we shouldn't just sit and wait for it to make the situation go away and return our lives to normal.

The Role of Nutrition

While the narrative we typically hear has offered vaccines as our best hope, the emerging puzzle pieces are telling a bigger story—one that gives nutrition a central role.

Ongoing research around vitamins D and K2 is pointing to why we as a global population are so susceptible to COVID-19. It's pointing to widespread nutritional deficiencies in vitamin D and vitamin K2 that affect our immune systems and our COVID-specific immune response.

Right now, the general feeling is that there's nothing we can do beyond trying to avoid the spread of germs. People feel they have no power. That's a wearying and stressful state to live in—and, from years of work as a physician, I know it also doesn't help your health. Most importantly, it's just not true.

We do have an element of control in making our bodies as powerful as we can through bringing attention to nutrition and living a healthier lifestyle.

You are less susceptible to infections of all kinds when you boost your immunity and decrease systemic inflammation in your body.

Specifically, we're finding that vitamins D and K2 may have the ability to help.

I see benefits to approaching the COVID-19 puzzle in a manner similar to my approach in my work as an infectious disease specialist. When studying infectious diseases, I look at the whole body. It all connects. Everything needs to be considered. To move through this pandemic and any new ones that rise, we need to look at everything we can do. We need to approach the pandemic holistically. This means masks, social distancing, exploring and utilizing treatments and vaccines, and also turning to nutrition.

Nutrition can't be left out.

Nutrition is also not a magic solution. What it is, though, is an added strategy that—unlike drugs with possible side effects—has very little potential to hurt but has great potential to help on a large scale. It's also a strategy that serves as a foundation to make the other interventions and recommendations work better. They all work together.

One remarkable advantage to this nutritional approach needs to be highlighted. When you decide to prioritize getting the nutrition you need—and specifically the vitamins D and K2—it creates a lasting foundation that extends into the future. Taking care of your body this way builds a foundation you can depend on and benefit from even after COVID, even when new viruses may arise.

The thought of new viruses might not be on your mind right now. Everyone wants to just get through this crisis. Things are supposed to go back to normal after it stops, right?

We do need to get through this particular crisis, and we'll be looking at what we are learning in the following chapters. However, the reality is that we've been due for a pandemic for decades, and it is almost certain that this won't be the last one. More and more viruses will emerge, and as a result of how we travel, once a virus appears somewhere, it quickly spreads everywhere. (COVID even made it to Antarctica.) When this does happen, we'll be starting from scratch in terms of research on the new viral disease.

It'll be important to dive into that research, but we need to improve the defenses we already have to truly change the situation. I don't believe that whenever a new virus appears, we should simply wait for the vaccine and treatments to be developed while people die. We are learning that we can take action with simple steps to build stronger immune systems so the next time a novel viral disease appears, things may look different.

We might be able to help prevent COVID-19 and other viruses from having such catastrophic effects by eating better, taking certain supplements when needed, and living a healthier lifestyle. This is a simple, logical, powerful approach we can take now and for the rest of our lives.

None of this replaces the treatments, vaccines, masks, and distancing—but nutrition and lifestyle are safe ways we can empower ourselves. You should absolutely be nourishing your immune health.

It's time to open this conversation and make changes.

In the medical community, we tend to look at drugs to solve problems. This goes back to our earliest training: we spend years on pharmacology and an average of 19 hours on nutrition. Writing that sentence seems shocking. In a four-year educational program that is designed to teach and train the primary healers of our society, we spend less than one week on nutrition. Physicians often come out of medical school with the opinion that vitamins aren't very important. It's true that one vitamin won't cure everything in the world, but to think they are nothing and not worth exploring? That's absurd.

In research, the emphasis is typically on drugs, too. As a researcher who's won a large number of National Institute of

Health (NIH) grants and as an NIH grant reviewer, I can tell you that studies investigating vitamins are much harder to get funded than studies around drugs. This is usually made clear right from the start in med school. Physicians know that if you want to do research and get funded, it's much easier to study a big biologic agent (a biological drug) with numerous effects. Those studies are certainly important and help many people; I do several of them in my work. However, not everyone is going to take that drug.

If you want to prevent diseases in large-scale populations, you ideally want a solution that is inexpensive, safe, and can be given on a large scale. This means we should be investing in well-done research on vitamins and supplements.

Our need to learn more about COVID-19 is now leading us into more of these studies.

It's a critical moment we're in, and the urgency of it offers a chance to reframe our approach to health. We need to use this crisis as a wake-up call to move from a reactionary mindset to a preventative one. In this book, we'll explore a preventative approach that nourishes your immune system with a specific focus on nutrition, and especially vitamins D and K2.

This preventative approach could benefit a vast number of people.

When most people think of poor immunity, they think of HIV or cancer, but there's a sizeable gray area between stellar immunity and the most serious immunodeficiency. Most people currently live in that gray zone, with less than optimal immunity that could be brought into a healthier range by making simple changes.

When your immune system is stronger, you have less inflammation in your body. Stronger immunity and decreased systemic inflammation have the potential to prevent both acute diseases like COVID-19 and also chronic diseases.

Strong immunity is power. Strong immunity can save and improve lives, and it depends on nutrition.

In the time of COVID-19, and what may be an age of pandemics, people need to understand the impact nutrition has on immunity and health. People need to understand what we're learning about vitamin D and vitamin K2.

This knowledge will change lives.

Let's start exploring it and spreading the knowledge.

CHAPTER 2

The Foundation for Strong Immunity

Most people don't tend to think much about nourishing their immune systems with nutrition and a healthy lifestyle—but we need to. Before we dive into discussion of the immune system and specific nutrients like vitamins D and K2, I want to spend some time discussing the idea of nutrition and lifestyle more generally.

Nutrient Deficiency Is Not a Thing of the Past

Supplying your body with good nutrition can be dramatically beneficial, and nutritional deficiency can be very damaging. This probably seems straightforward enough to most people. But how we think about nutrition is often limited.

It's easy to assume nutritional deficiency isn't a big problem anymore when there's access to enough food. It's true people used to get diseases like scurvy (the result of severe vitamin C deficiency) that we rarely see anymore, at least in the

Western world. An important point I want to make is that adequate (or sufficient, for a better term) nutrition is about more than getting the bare minimum of a vitamin.

Nutrition is integral to every process your body does, and it's easy to become deficient in nutrients you need.

Dr. Myers has spent most of his professional life exploring the subject of nutrition and nutritional deficiency, and I find his perspective a valuable frame for discussion. Nutritional biochemistry can be quite complex, but as Dr. Myers notes, we don't need to understand all of the biochemical reactions happening in our bodies for them to happen. They function naturally. They do what they're designed to do without any input from us, except for in a few key areas. One of the most important of these is nutrition.

What is the simplest and most basic nutrient? Oxygen. We need a near-constant supply. We can only survive a matter of minutes without it.

Next in importance is water. Our bodies are 70 percent water, and we can only survive a few days without taking in more.

Then come the nutrients in food. What generally receives the most attention today are the *macro*nutrients—proteins, fats, and carbohydrates. But just like nutrition is about more than avoiding scurvy, it's also about more than the proteins, fats, and carbohydrates that dominate most diet books. Of course your body needs these things, but what's equally important is that it gets a wide, steady supply of *micro*nutrients. These are the vitamins, minerals, trace minerals, and other accessory nutrients and phytonutrients your body needs to function at its best. By best, I don't mean at the level of an Olympic athlete. I mean functioning well enough to do all the processes they're meant to do to help you stay healthy.

The Importance of Vitamins

Scientific awareness of vitamins and micronutrients is relatively recent, developing from the work of Casimir Funk in the early 20th century.

Before that, 19th-century nutritional dogma advanced the idea that a healthy diet was comprised of only four components: protein, mineral, fat, and carbohydrate. When research by Funk and his colleagues showed that animals fed only these four things failed to thrive, they realized something else must be missing. This realization was corroborated by research around the diseases beri-beri and scurvy, which researchers discovered could be prevented by specific substances beyond the categories of protein, mineral, fat, or carbohydrate.

Funk proposed that there were "vital amines"—amines being a type of chemical compound—present in foods that were needed for survival. He named these necessary substances by combining the words into "vitamine." And while it was later discovered that these necessary nutrients weren't limited to the single structural category of amines, a form of the original name stuck.[1]

1. DeLuca, H.F. "History of the Discovery of Vitamin D and Its Active Metabolites," *BoneKEy Reports*, January 8, 2014, 3: 479. https://www. ncbi.nlm.nih.gov/pmc/articles/PMC3899558/

Almost every function of the body depends on micronutrients.

Micronutrients act as building blocks for our cells and cofactors for our enzymes, and they are the functional components of almost every activity in the body.

Without enough micronutrients, things don't function as well. This affects every system in the body, including the immune system. Dr. Myers refers to this faltering functionality as the *3D Effect*, the three stages of what he calls nutrient deficiency syndrome (NDS).

When the body doesn't receive the essential nutrients it needs—again, a situation that is still common today, even in developed countries—a process begins that leads to dysfunction. Once this dysfunction becomes visible enough, we tend to then label the resulting symptoms as a disease. Typically, though, the body had one or more issues prior to diagnosis. The body developed a diseased state after first going through various stages of deficiency that eventually reached a point where they became easier to recognize (and probably more difficult to live with).

The first stage of nutrient deficiency is depletion. This happens when the body isn't receiving one or more essential nutrients at the level one or more systems need to function optimally. Any stores the body has are then utilized to make up the difference.

The second stage is deficiency. The body reaches this stage when chronic depletion of one or more essential nutrients initiates a breakdown of body systems at the cellular level.

The third stage is dysfunction. This happens when enough cellular damage has occurred that the breakdown of body systems manifests as visible symptoms. When these symptoms cluster in recognizable patterns at high enough levels, they get labeled as a particular disease.

The disease deserves treatment and care of course, but it's important to realize the earlier two stages of this process also deserve attention. There's a nutritional problem long before the body reaches the point of official disease diagnosis. We don't want to wait to get to dysfunction to address it.

Nutrient Deficiency Syndrome Progress

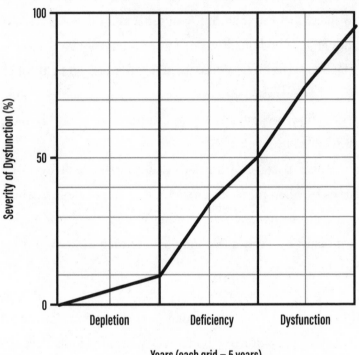

Years (each grid = 5 years)

The three stages of the nutrient deficiency syndrome. From Ignarro, Louis, Ph.D., and Andrew Myers, N.D. *Health Is Wealth: 10 Power Nutrients That Increase Your Odds of Living to 100* (Health Value Publications, 2009), p. 51. Used with permission.

Addressing nutritional deficiencies earlier makes a re-markable difference because this is an accelerating process that can easily become a damaging cascade. When you enter a depletion stage for one nutrient, that specific depletion re-quires the body to compensate by using more of other nutrients. Often, this leads to other nutrients then becoming depleted. In this way, it can turn into a merciless, compounding cycle that causes damage at the cellular level.

So the question becomes, how do we take in sufficient amounts of vital nutrients to avoid falling into depletion in the first place?

Reframe Your View of "Diet"

As you probably would imagine, we start taking in the necessary nutrients through daily food choices—what is often called diet. The word "diet," though, is somewhat problematic because it reflects part of why we're in this situation, where a large number of people are depleted in nutrients.

Our culture uses this word a lot. We all know we're supposed to eat a healthy diet. Most people understand the word in this context to mean our daily food choices, rather than the short-term change it can also refer to, one usually focused on weight loss and cutting certain foods out. But I would argue that the connotation of cutting things out is still wrapped up in the term "diet" and a misdirected perception about healthy eating.

Often people tend to associate a healthy diet with *not* eating certain foods. There's some truth to this. Removing or cutting out certain foods can be great for your health. Take added sugar, which most frequently in the U.S. means high-fructose corn syrup. There's nothing about this substance that helps your body. When I cut it out of my own diet, I lost about 12 pounds—without doing anything else. Additionally, there are foods that can be healthy or neutral for some bodies, but interact with other bodies in ways that impair health. Of course we want to be aware of this and try to avoid foods that cause problems for us.

Yet when your idea of a healthy diet so thoroughly focuses around what you're trying to keep out, it's easy to forget about what you need to take in. Many people seem to think that avoiding foods they view as problematic while eating anything else is good enough.

It is good enough to keep you from starvation. Yet it won't nourish your body in a way that keeps your immunity, or any other system, strong. To do that, you need to think about the foods you *are* eating as much as the ones you aren't. From there, you need to go beyond the macronutrients that dominate food labels and public conversation and bring your attention to micronutrients, like vitamins and minerals.

To get all the micronutrients your body needs to be healthy, you need to take in plenty of micronutrients through your daily food choices. I'll talk in more detail about how to do this in the final chapter on putting everything together.

For guidance on what to eat every day, I love to start with the Harvard Healthy Eating Pyramid.[2]

---

2. "Healthy Eating Pyramid," *The Nutrition Source*, Harvard T.H. Chan School of Public Health, accessed January 15, 2021: https://www.hsph.harvard.edu/nutritionsource/healthy-eating-pyramid/

Use the Harvard Healthy Eating Pyramid guidelines to help you choose more micronutrient-rich foods.

It's important to put more emphasis on fresh produce as the core of your daily diet, and while whole grains are nutrient rich, you need more diverse sources of micronutrients than grains provide. The Harvard Healthy Eating Pyramid places vegetables and fruits, along with healthy fats and oils and whole grains, at the foundation of a healthy diet. While it's important to note that not everyone tolerates grains well and this is something you may want to adjust, this pyramid is generally a great approach—and a valuable shift from the standard pyramid we're used to seeing, which places whole grains alone at the foundation.

Placing fruits and vegetables at the base of your diet means you're likely taking in a variety of micronutrients through your food. This is critical, and your body will thank you. As we think about nutrition as the foundation of strong immunity, it's still important to ask, though, are these foods enough to give us the nutrients we need?

Supplementation Is the Beneficial Boost You Almost Always Need

In ideal conditions, healthy daily food choices would be enough to nourish ourselves with adequate nutrition. The reality, though, is that our modern lives are demanding in ways that tax the body and increase our nutritional needs. Many of us live with chronic stress and almost all of us, even when we try to minimize our exposure, are surrounded by a level of environmental toxins that place additional burdens on our bodies. To cope with these factors, our bodies need to take in more micronutrients than ever. Yet while we need more of them, modern agriculture practices have actually led to depleted soil that produces less nutritious food. When I say less nutritious food, I mean substantially, even shockingly less.

Studies have shown that fruits and vegetables today have up to 40 percent fewer vitamins and minerals than they did 50 years ago.[3]

---

3. Davis, D.R., M.D. Epp, and H.D. Riordan. "Changes in USDA Food Composition Data for 43 Garden Crops, 1950 to 1999," *Journal of the American College of Nutrition*, December 2004, 23(6): 669-82. https://pubmed.ncbi. nlm.nih.gov/15637215/; Davis, D.R. "Declining Fruit and Vegetable Nutrient Composition: What Is the Evidence?" *Hort. Science*, February 2009, 44(1): 15-19. https://journals.ashs.org/hortsci/view/journals/hortsci/44/1/article-p15.xml

At the same time, the Western diet is also surprisingly sparse in certain key micronutrients. Unfortunately, this is particularly true when it comes to vitamin K2 and vitamin D.

Eating fresh food is still important and a cornerstone of good health—I can't emphasis this enough—but it's unlikely to be sufficient on its own, even with a seemingly perfect diet. Many of us don't eat that seemingly perfect diet anyway.

This is where supplementation can help. It reflects the reality of modern life and what we need. (And for this reason, I'm pleased to see it included in the Harvard Healthy Eating Pyramid.)

Dr. Myers and I use supplements for our own health, and I encourage everyone I know to do the same. By identifying the most vital micronutrients for your body and then taking them regularly in supplement form, you fill in possible gaps in your nutrition and better enable your systems to work as they're meant to.

There's a lot more to say here. As we continue, we'll talk more specifically about some of these gaps and how they affect your immune system. Our focus in this book remains on vitamins D and K2 but in the final chapter, we'll also look at other supplements you might want to consider.

Lifestyle Habits Matter

I don't want to spend too much time stating what may seem obvious, but lifestyle choices beyond nutrition also make a huge difference in your health and immunity.

When I talk about lifestyle choices, I mean all the things that you do over and over in your day that contribute to what's going on in your body. This can cover hundreds of behaviors, many of which can affect your immune system negatively or positively.

Some of the most critical things that support your immune system are sleep, regular physical activity, and finding healthy ways to manage stress. (I'll get into more on these topics later.)

Some of the things that damage or stress our immune systems are eating too much sugar, drinking alcohol, and smoking.

First, let's talk about sugar. Earlier, I emphasized what we need to take in. Yet it would be irresponsible to not also touch on this one substance, sugar, that wreaks such havoc on your body. Sugar has significant and unhealthy effects: it can lead to inflammation, insulin resistance, cancer, weight gain, and other dysfunctions. It's also a problem for your immune system.

Eating 20 teaspoons of sugar per day can suppress the body's immune response, and unfortunately, many of us routinely eat this amount—and more.[4]

4. "Harmful Effects of Excess Sugar," AskDrSears.com: https://www.askdrsears.com/topics/feeding-eating/family-nutrition/sugar/harmful-effects-excess-sugar

Today, the average American consumes almost 152 pounds of sugar in one year. This is equal to three pounds (or six cups) of sugar consumed a week. That's almost a cup of sugar each day.[5] Since one cup of sugar is equivalent to 48 teaspoons of sugar, the average American is eating more than twice the amount that has negative effects on immunity.

Another significant factor that can weaken immune health is alcohol intake. While studies about the benefits of a glass of red wine consistently make the news, and some people seem to think you can help knock out a bug with a hot toddy, the reality is that alcohol depresses your immune system. The World Health Organization (WHO) recently stated, "Alcohol consumption is associated with a range of communicable and noncommunicable diseases and mental health disorders, which can make a person more vulnerable to COVID-19. In particular, alcohol compromises the body's immune system and increases the risk of adverse health outcomes."[6] When you're seeking to improve your immune health, it's best to avoid alcohol entirely or minimize your intake.

Smoking hurts your body in several critical ways, and that includes weakening your immune system and increasing inflammation.

5. "How Much Sugar Do You Eat? You May Be Surprised," New Hampshire Department of Health and Human Services: https://www.dhhs.nh.gov/dphs/nhp/documents/sugar.pdf

6. Ries, Julia. "How Alcohol Can Affect Your Immune System," *Healthline*, April 22, 2020: https://www.healthline.com/health-news/can-alcohol-hurt-your-immune-system-during-COVID-19-outbreak

If you needed one more reason to quit, your immune health, both in and out of the pandemic, is a good one.

I realize that lifestyle choices can be difficult changes to make and sustain, especially in the middle of periods of additional stress. However, I encourage you to seriously try to make healthy choices in these areas if you don't already. Unhealthy lifestyle choices are at the root of many health problems—to the extent that one-fourth of U.S. healthcare costs are attributed to modifiable lifestyle factors.[7]

It doesn't have to be this way.

As you try to make changes, be patient with yourself but also keep moving in a healthier direction. Know that in making an effort here, you're giving yourself a gift. As these healthy lifestyle choices support your immunity, they can also support your mental well-being and all aspects of your health. During a pandemic, that's even more important. I hope this chapter has made clear how deeply nutrition and healthy lifestyle choices are needed to support every system of the body. Now that we have this context, let's zoom in on the primary topic we want to explore: the immune system.

---

7. Wooldridge, Scott. "Changing Lifestyle Choices Could Cut $730B in Annual Health Care Spending," *BenefitsPRO*, October 5, 2020: https://www.benefitspro.com/2020/10/05/changing-lifestyle-choices-could-cut-730b-in-annual-health-care-spending/

CHAPTER 3

Understanding the Immune System

Since supporting your immunity is essential to protecting your health during this pandemic and beyond, I want to explore this process in some detail. There's a lot of technical information in this chapter, but it's useful to understand.

The COVID-19 pandemic has brought the importance of immune health into the public eye. We have an opportunity to move into a more preventative approach regarding our health. Prevention has not been our default mode, as a healthcare system or as individuals. Part of that is a systemic problem, and part of that seems to be our human nature: we often just don't want to make changes before we're forced to.

For example, in my work with HIV patients, bone health is often an important concern, and a variety of studies, including some of my own, have shown vitamin D can significantly help. I recently told a patient with low vitamin D she should start taking D daily to get her levels up, but she didn't take that step. It didn't feel like enough of a worry to do something differently. Then, eventually, her bones started showing visible damage. Now she's taking the vitamin D. It's still beneficial for her at this later stage and I'm glad she's taking it, but starting sooner almost certainly would have helped her more.

Prevention is pivotal. Yet as a healthcare system and as individuals, we so often discount it.

And I get it. When we're told to change habits to prevent something that might not happen anyway, it doesn't exactly trigger the pleasure centers in our brains. There's often little motivation to make the change. The level of urgency involved isn't the same as when you're confronted with a serious diagnosis that scares you into feeling you need to change something immediately.

The pandemic is a situation that falls in the middle. Getting sick from COVID-19 feels like a more imminent possibility for many of us than the idea of possibly getting heart disease down the road, maybe a decade or more into the future. The pandemic situation may motivate us to look for preventative actions we can take to care for our bodies.

But some of the things we're learning that might help, like ensuring healthy levels of vitamins D and K2, are easy to do and require relatively little of us. It can be as simple as taking a couple of supplements each day.

Yet even such a simple, easy action as taking a supplement requires you to act in some way—perhaps in a slightly different way than you have before. You need to overcome some inertia to begin something—to open a webpage to order a supplement or write it down on your shopping list. Then you may need to develop a new routine to make taking the supplement part of your day. Getting past that inertia is necessary, even for what's essentially the easiest thing you can do for your immune health. Other lifestyle factors that are also vital to your health and immunity take more effort and bigger changes.

I want to explore the immune system in depth because the more you know about how your immune system works and the role nutrients play in that process, the more motivation you'll likely have to adopt preventative habits. Understanding the deep need for nutrients makes them matter more, and that can motivate our behaviors.

So let's begin.

How the Immune System Works

Let's start by looking at the immune system in general.

What does this system do, exactly?

The immune system is the body's natural protection against invaders—harmful microorganisms like bacteria and viruses. Put another way, the immune system is a defensive resource that's there to protect you, and its presence gives you freedom to explore the world.

The stronger your immune function is, the better equipped your body is to fight infection and disease.

As we've already touched on, a person's immunity varies based on some key characteristics such as individual's genetics, lifestyle, environmental factors, age, and nutrition. It peaks around age 20 and then gradually begins to decline from there. Genetics and age are beyond our control, but many other factors aren't—and I truly can't overstate this.

Immune response draws upon a wide variety of cells for many functions, involving both nonspecific (innate) components and specific (adaptive) components, all of which are closely linked and work together.

Innate and Adaptive Immune Response

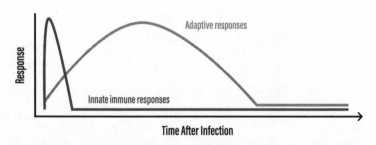

Typical innate and adaptive immune responses as an infection progresses.

The innate immune response is made up of nonspecific components. These components of the immune system defend against infections in general rather than against specific threats. These include barriers like skin that prevent invaders from entering the body in the first place, and eliminators, which are cells and chemicals that stop invaders from spreading. These nonspecific components are naturally present.

Innate immune responses are immediate, peak quickly, and then fall. Cells involved in an innate immune response include neutrophils, monocytes/macrophages, natural killer (NK) cells, and complement proteins.

The adaptive immune response, on the other hand, is made of specific components. These involve cells that are specially adapted to a particular threat. They are pathogen-specific and learned or developed after exposure. They are known as adaptive, or acquired, immunity. When the adaptive immune system is triggered by a pathogen for the first time, the immune response builds more slowly. Cells involved in an adaptive immune response include T-cells and B-cells. These cells are types of white blood cells, which are produced in the bone marrow.

The immune system is activated by antigens, which are substances the body recognizes as foreign. Antigens commonly include proteins found on bacteria, fungi, and viruses.

How is an autoimmune disease different?

As a side note, I want to mention that the immune system can also be activated by proteins on its own cells when it mistakes these proteins for foreign substances. When this happens, it's known as an autoimmune response. While this can be a significant health concern, it's a different immune response than what we mean when we refer to the response that helps our bodies prevent or fight off infectious disease.

Now let's look more closely at what happens when the immune system encounters a virus. Again, we're going to need to get a little more technical as we lay this scientific groundwork. Bear with me.

The Immune Response to Viruses

When a virus enters the body, it first triggers an innate (non-specific) response. Viruses are adaptable and often good at avoiding detection as they replicate, but when NK cells discover virally infected cells, they release toxic substances that kill them. Often, a virus is controlled by this innate immune response. But when it isn't—meaning that it replicates faster than the innate system can clear it—then the body moves into an adaptive (specific) response.

At this point, communication is needed between the innate and adaptive systems. This communication is carried out by cytokines and by cell-to-cell interactions between dendritic cells, T-cells, and B-cells. B-cells become the cells that produce antibodies, and T-cells recognize and kill virus-infected cells. Subsets of both B-cells and T-cells preserve memory of the virus, which enables a much faster response to the same virus in the future. The effectiveness of the adaptive response determines whether the infection is cleared.

An uncontrolled adaptive response—for example, a toxic cytokine storm, something you may have heard about in connection to COVID-19—can cause damage of its own.

What are cytokines?

Cytokines are small proteins that act as signaling molecules between cells in the body. While the first cytokine wave begins during the innate immune response, cytokines are also produced during the body's adaptive immune response. It's during an uncontrolled adaptive response that the cytokine response can become dangerous and tip into a toxic cytokine storm, in which the body starts to attack tissues and cells not related to the virus.

The Immune Response to COVID-19

Let's now look closely at COVID-19.

The COVID-19 disease moves through the body in up to four phases: the incubation phase, symptomatic phase, early pulmonary phase, and systemic inflammation phase.

Immunopathology of COVID-19: How the Body Responds

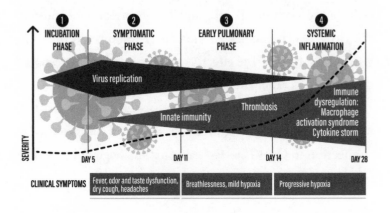

The four phases of COVID-19 infection related to appearance of clinical symptoms and immune response.

When COVID first enters the body, it moves through the incubation phase, where the virus utilizes proteins called ACE2 receptors to enter the cells and begin replicating. The length of this phase can potentially last up to 14 days, but most commonly lasts two to four days.

Next, the disease progresses into the symptomatic phase. Here, virus replication continues as the body begins its innate immune response, which includes the first cytokine wave. In this phase, the patient may feel symptoms including fever, fatigue, loss of smell and taste, dry cough, and headaches. The length of the symptomatic phase varies from patient to patient. In this stage, the disease will begin to improve or resolve fully, or the infection will progress.

If the virus continues to advance, it will next move into the early pulmonary phase. Here, the patient may experience breathlessness and mild hypoxia, where regions of the body are deprived of the oxygen they need at the tissue level. This is also the period where thrombosis—another term for a clot in a blood vessel—may set in.

From this point, the patient may move into systemic inflammation. In this stage, they may experience progressive hypoxia, with the body being deprived of oxygen in even more damaging ways. This stage holds the risk of a harmful cytokine storm, which can sometimes lead to acute respiratory distress syndrome (ARDS). Downstream effects from here can include thrombosis, septic shock, and multi-organ failure. I probably don't need to tell you that this is a dangerous stage to be in.

The death tolls we've seen headlining the news are typically related to the virus entering this fourth phase of systemic inflammation. The third stage also holds significant dangers from thrombosis.

Reaching either the third or the fourth stages is a real possibility whether you know you're at risk (that is, you have a comorbidity) or not. Clearly there are still unknown risk factors we need to understand.

Yet as we know, it's also true that many people who are exposed never get sick. In these people, the innate immune response defeats the virus. Another significant group of people who experience symptoms (the symptomatic phase) never progress beyond the second stage. Again, the body's immune defenses are able to conquer the virus at this second stage. The virus can take a devastating path, but whether it does so has often seemed unpredictable.

Nutritional Deficiency Affects the Immune Response

While many unknowns remain as to why some people have much more severe cases of COVD-19 than others, we're learning more about what may be behind some of this seeming unpredictability. We're learning how significant a role nutrients and nutritional deficiency can play.

As we've mentioned, nutrients are needed for all the systems in your body, and when you don't get enough of even one nutrient, you can start seeing depletion, deficiency, and dysfunction.

A variety of amino acids, minerals, and vitamins are essential to the immune system. The body needs these nutrients to create new immune cells, messenger substances, and antibodies. And just like with other systems, when even one of these nutrients isn't available in the right quantity at the time the body needs it, the immune system can't work properly.

Some of the most vital building blocks the immune system needs include lysine, taurine, zinc, selenium, and vitamins A, C, E, D, and K2. Many of these are widely known for their role in supporting general immunity, but vitamins

D and K2 have more recently gained the attention of the medical and research community. The growing body of research is compelling.

Vitamin D has a significant role in the immune system—the system simply can't activate without it. Without sufficient vitamin D, the T-cells remain dormant and can do nothing to fight serious infections.[8] Vitamin D is even known as the "antibiotic vitamin" due to its anti-inflammatory, immune-regulating effect.[9]

When we look at how vitamin D affects viruses in particular, the evidence is striking.

A three-year clinical study discovered that the intake of vitamin D significantly reduced the occurrence of influenza and colds, and even brought winter infection numbers down to match that of summer.[10] And according to a large meta-analysis based on 25 double-blind studies with over 11,000

8. von Essen, M.R., Martin Kongsbak, Peter Schjerling, Klaus Olgaard, Niels Ødum, and Carsten Geisler. "Vitamin D Controls T Cell Antigen Receptor Signaling and Activation of Human T Cells," *Nature Immunology*, 2010, 11: 344–349. https://www.nature.com/articles/ni.1851

9. Schauber, Jürgen, et al. "Injury Enhances TLR2 Function and Antimicrobial Peptide Expression through a Vitamin D-Dependent Mechanism," *Journal of Clinical Investigation*, 2007, 117(3): 803–811. https://pubmed.ncbi.nlm.nih. gov/17290304/; Raloff, J. "The Antibiotic Vitamin," *Science News*, 2006, 170: 312–17. https://onlinelibrary.wiley.com/doi/10.2307/4017406; Zasloff, M. "Inducing Endogenous Antimicrobial Peptides to Battle Infections," *Proceedings of the National Academy of Sciences of the USA*, 2006, 103(24): 8913–14. https:// www.ncbi.nlm.nih.gov/pmc/articles/PMC1482538/

10. Aloia, J., and M. Li-Ng. "Re: Epidemic Influenza and Vitamin D," *Epidemiology & Infection*, 2007, 135(7): 1095–1096. https://pubmed.ncbi.nlm. nih.gov/17352842/

study participants, vitamin D supplementation reduced the risk of acute respiratory disease by up to 70 percent in people with a low vitamin D output status.[11]

What is a meta-analysis?

A meta-analysis is a statistical analysis that combines the results of several independent but related studies. Bringing this data together helps researchers better evaluate it and make conclusions.

With vitamin K2, we don't currently have clear evidence of it impacting the immune system in general to the same extent as vitamin D. What we do know, though, is that it has a positive effect on inflammation, which could contribute to a healthy immune inflammatory response.

A 2016 paper on the role of vitamin K in chronic aging diseases stated that in vitro ("in vitro" means in a test tube or other simulated environment, not in a living system) and animal experiments have determined that vitamin K suppressed production of pro-inflammatory cytokines. The paper also noted that higher vitamin K intake has been associated with

11. Martineau, A.R., et al. "Vitamin D Supplementation to Prevent Acute Respiratory Tract Infections: Systematic Review and Meta-Analysis of Individual Participant Data," *BMJ*, 2017, 356: i6583. https://www.bmj.com/content/356/bmj.i6583

lower inflammation overall and with lower concentrations of several individual pro-inflammatory biomarkers.[12]

Inflammation is both a hero and a villain in the body. Our immune cells use inflammatory chemical mediators to destroy viruses and bacteria; it's a powerful, necessary tool. However, if it gets out of control, it can cause problems. Vitamin K2 can help to keep inflammation under control. It helps stop the generalized reaction and in addition, it also turns off other inflammatory chemical mediators throughout the body. Without this, the body can't regulate and control a healthy immune response.

How Nutritional Deficiency Affects the COVID-19 Immune Response

Now it gets really interesting.

Let's quickly look at how deficiencies in vitamins D and K2 seem to be intersecting with COVID-19. There's a lot of research on this and we'll get into much more of it later. For now, we'll just touch on two studies for brief context—just to get a sense of how research points toward vitamin D and vitamin K2 deficiencies being connected to worse COVID outcomes—before returning to look at the disease's progression throughout the body.

---

12. Harshman, Stephanie G., and M. Kyla Shea. "The Role of Vitamin K in Chronic Aging Diseases: Inflammation, Cardiovascular Disease, and Osteoarthritis," *Current Nutrition Reports*, June 2016, 5(2): 90–98. https://www. ncbi.nlm.nih.gov/pmc/articles/PMC5026413/

A meta-analysis on vitamin D that included over 8,000 COVID-19 patients participating in 26 studies observed that people with severe COVID were shown to have 65 percent greater vitamin D deficiency compared to those with a milder prognosis.[13]

A recent study on vitamin K suggested that vitamin K deficiency in COVID patients may increase pro-inflammatory cytokines that could support the dangerous cytokine storm. Deficiency in this essential vitamin can also "contribute to those events involved in vascular calcification leading to thrombosis and disseminate intravascular coagulation (DIC), which feature the microvascular damage observed in COVID-19 patients."[14]

We can see why these deficiencies may have such an effect on COVID-19 outcomes when we return to the journey of the virus through the body, and identify vitamin D's and vitamin K2's modes of action along the way.

Let's start once again when the virus first enters the body in the incubation phase. This is when the virus uses ACE2 receptors and other coreceptors to enter the cells. Vitamin D

13. Pereira, Marcos, Alialdo Dantas Damascena, Laylla Mirella Galvão Azevedo, Tarcio de Almeida Oliveira, and Jerusa da Mota Santana. "Vitamin D Deficiency Aggravates COVID-19: Systematic Review and Meta-Analysis," *Critical Reviews in Food Science and Nutrition*, November 4, 2020: 1-9. https://doi.org/10.1080/1 0408398.2020.1841090. https://pubmed.ncbi.nlm.nih.gov/33146028/

14. Anastasi, Emanuela, Cristiano Ialongo, Raffaella Labriola, Giampiero Ferraguti, Marco Lucarelli, and Antonio Angeloni. "Vitamin K Deficiency and COVID-19," *Scandinavian Journal of Clinical and Laboratory Investigation*, 2020, 80(6): 1-3. https://doi.org/10.1080/00365513.2020.1805122

downregulates the expression of these receptors (in a sense, turns them off) that are so necessary to the virus, which means the virus has less opportunity to take root. Here, vitamin D is supporting the body's immediate innate response; it also goes on to support the body's adaptive response.

Throughout the whole process, but most importantly during the early incubation and early symptomatic phases, vitamins D and K2 downregulate the NF-kB signaling pathways—which are needed to trigger inflammation—and secretion of cytokines, helping to avoid the toxic cytokine storm. Vitamin K2 is also valuable in these later stages of the virus, as it's used to activate proteins involved in the prevention of thrombosis and soft tissue calcification.

What is NF-kB?

NF-kB stands for "nuclear factor-kappaB" and refers to a family of transcription factors that have important roles in the coordination of genes that control immune responses. They are the subject of research into understanding the regulation and function of the immune response as it relates to cancer and other diseases.

Vitamin D's and Vitamin K2's Roles During the Progression of COVID-19

Vitamin D downregulates the expression of ACE2 receptors. This downregulation gives the virus less opportunity to take root.

Vitamins D *and* K2 downregulate the NF-kB signaling pathways that are needed to trigger inflammation and secretion of cytokines, which helps to prevent a cytokine storm.

Vitamin K2 activates proteins that prevent thrombosis and soft tissue calcification, which means it helps protect lungs and the vascular system.

It's clear that vitamins D and K2 are important players in slowing or stopping the progression of this virus. They're also important players in our overall immune function.

Now that we've looked at how the immune system works, we've followed the path of COVID-19 through the body, and we've seen how vitamins D and K2 intersect with both the immune system and the COVID disease progression, we're ready to unfold another layer. Next, let's go deeper into the research around vitamins D and K2.

CHAPTER 4

The Pivotal Roles of Vitamin D

I'm passionate about research, as you have probably gathered by now, so I'm excited to get into this chapter. We're in a thrilling moment with vitamins D and K2—especially K2, around which new understandings are beginning to take clear shape.

It's amazing to me to think how we can go from knowing almost nothing about something to realizing how essential it's always been. Once we learn about a vital process or substance and come to understand how significant it is, it can seem almost crazy to think there was a point when we didn't realize it.

We might be at that point with vitamin K2. We've known the importance of vitamin D longer, but our understanding there is also still relatively new. It's incredible what we've learned about both—and what we are still uncovering.

While this book focuses on immune health, it's important to touch on a range of things we've discovered and are discovering around vitamins D and K2. First, their function in different systems helps us better understand how we should use them to support our immunity. Second, because I am a whole-body physician, the roles we are discovering for these vitamins help to fill gaps in knowledge for a clearer understanding of how those roles are connected to other body systems. Since most of this information hasn't been talked or written about much, I want to give you the chance to hear at least a piece of the wider story, including their histories.

We can credit vitamin D's discovery to work done to investigate rickets, a disorder that leads to the softening and weakening of bones in children. While rickets can be genetic or tied to other deficiencies, it's most often the result of severe vitamin D deficiency.

Rickets was a common disease in 17th-century England and continued to affect children in the U.S. and Europe up through the late 19th century and early 20th century. At that time, there was a significant expansion in knowledge regarding the disease, stemming from observations made as a result of animal dietary experiments with cod-liver oil and irradiation of food, both of which cured rickets. When vitamin A was removed from the cod-liver oil, a new vitamin, called vitamin D, was credited with the effect on the disease. The vitamin's structure was identified in 1932.[15]

---

15. DeLuca, H.F. "History of the Discovery of Vitamin D and Its Active Metabolites," *BoneKEy Reports*, January 8, 2014, 3: 479. https://www.ncbi.nlm. nih.gov/pmc/articles/PMC3899558/

The Well-Known Benefits of Vitamin D

Vitamin D is currently best known for its role in bone and cardiovascular health and the immune system.

Calcium is what first comes to mind when most people think of bone health, yet calcium on its own isn't enough to support the bones. For calcium to reach the bones, the body must go through a few processes that rely on vitamin D—as well as vitamin K2, which we'll learn about next. Vitamin D transports calcium from the gut through the intestinal wall and into the blood stream, where it can then be available for bones. Vitamin D is also necessary for the synthesis of osteocalcin and matrix Gla protein, both of which are needed to bring calcium from the bloodstream into the bones.

I've been working in HIV research around vitamin D for a decade and I've seen firsthand the protective and building effects it has on bone health in both adults and children with HIV.

Evidence also suggests vitamin D plays an important role in heart health. Low vitamin D levels are associated with hypertension, cardiovascular diseases and risk factors, and all-cause mortality.[16]

---

16. Kheiri, Babikir, Ahmed Abdalla, Mohammed Osman, Sahar Ahmed, Mustafa Hassan, and Ghassan Bachuwa. "Vitamin D Deficiency and Risk of Cardiovascular Diseases: A Narrative Review," *Clinical Hypertension*, 2018, 24: 9. https://www.ncbi.nlm.nih.gov/pmc/articles/PMC6013996/

Osteocalcin (OCN): Osteocalcin is a protein present in bones that is produced by osteoblasts (cells that form bone tissue). It is involved in the process of bone mineralization. Osteocalcin levels are generally considered a marker of bone formation. Its activation is dependent on vitamin K2 and stimulated by vitamin D.

Matrix Gla protein (MGP): Matrix Gla protein is a protein involved in inhibiting vascular calcification and promoting bone formation. Like osteocalcin, its production is dependent on vitamin K2 and stimulated by vitamin D.

Vitamin D also plays an essential role in the immune system as part of both innate and adaptive immunity. In innate immunity, vitamin D has been shown to offer protection against a number of infections and help modulate the immune system. In adaptive immunity, vitamin D seems to have a beneficial effect on T-cells and B-cells.[17] In my HIV research, we've seen this borne out as well, finding that vitamin D supplementation in youth with HIV not only increased their bone density but also improved their innate and adaptive immunity.

In terms of viral defense, vitamin D is gaining increasing recognition. A 2013 study of 5,660 participants found that

---

17. Siddiqui, Maheen, Judhell S. Manansala, Hana A. Abdulrahman, Gheyath K. Nasrallah, Maria K. Smatti, Nadin Younes, Asmaa A. Althani, and Hadi M. Yassine. "Immune Modulatory Effects of Vitamin D on Viral Infections," *Nutrients*, 2020 12(9): 2879. https://www.ncbi.nlm.nih.gov/pmc/articles/PMC7551809/

vitamin D decreased the risk of respiratory tract infections,[18] and a 2017 study extended this conclusion to indicate that vitamin D decreased the risk of acute respiratory tract infection by 70 percent.[19] Then in 2019, 24 studies, 19 of which were meta-analyses, found that serum vitamin D levels (measured in the blood) were inversely associated with the risk and severity of acute respiratory tract infections.[20] An inverse association means more vitamin D in the blood correlated with better outcomes—that is, reduced incidence and severity.

This is pretty significant data, and it leads us to COVID-19. As I mentioned earlier, my research team at U.H. in Cleveland went straight to work as soon as we heard of the disease beginning to spread in China. So did other researchers around the world.

Scientific studies are officially published after completing a lengthy peer-review process, but before this happens, versions are publicly shared as preprints. Usually these

18. Bergman, Peter, Åsa U. Lindh, Linda Björkhem-Bergman, and Jonatan D. Lindh. "Vitamin D and Respiratory Tract Infections: A Systematic Review and Meta-Analysis of Randomized Controlled Trials," *PLOS One*, 2013, 8(6): 0065835. https://journals.plos.org/plosone/article?id=10.1371/journal.pone.0065835

19. Martineau, A.R., et al. "Vitamin D Supplementation to Prevent Acute Respiratory Tract Infections: Systematic Review and Meta-Analysis of Individual Participant Data," *BMJ*, 2017, 356: i6583. https://www.bmj.com/content/356/bmj.i6583

20. Pham, Hai, Aninda Rahman, Azam Majidi, Mary Waterhouse, and Rachel E. Neale. "Acute Respiratory Tract Infection and 25-Hydroxyvitamin D Concentration: A Systematic Review and Meta-Analysis," *International Journal of Environmental Research and Public Health*, 2019, 16(17): 3020. https://www.mdpi.com/1660-4601/16/17/3020/htm

preprints don't enter public or media discussion, but with people all around the world dying, emerging data related to COVID-19 outcomes drew substantial amounts of interest and attention, which sparked further studies.

Some of those studies have investigated vitamin D. Let's walk through some of what researchers have discovered so far.

Who's Behind a Clinical Research Study?

When people picture a study, they sometimes imagine a few dedicated researchers spending all their time doing experiments in a lab—but a lot more goes on than that.

A clinical research study involves many diverse moving parts and needs a broad set of people. In my hospital system, we have several core groups that each contribute greatly to a study and help ensure the safety of study participants and the integrity of our final data.

A clinical research study is led by a *principal investigator* (P.I.), usually an M.D. but sometimes a Ph.D., who acts as the overall responsible party and reviews the work of the entire team. The P.I. usually has other physicians helping them, along with nurses and coordinators. Together, they make up the clinical core of the study. As you'd expect, this group includes the people who meet with the patients participating in the study.

We also have a *financial core*, staff who ensure that when a study is sponsored by someone else, the hospital gets paid just the right amount—otherwise, it could appear the hospital is either financially benefiting from the study or subsidizing a for-profit company. The financial core people handle these considerations, along with budgets, legal contracts, and billing.

Then there's the *regulatory core*. They handle patient consent and communication with regulatory departments and local hospital departments. The regulatory core documents everything throughout the entire process and does a lot of work behind the scenes to ensure all data is correct and transferrable to the FDA (the U.S. Food and Drug Administration).

Study samples go out to either the hospital clinical lab or a research lab that runs a specific type of assay, depending on the study needs. We also have our own pharmacy for research, the Investigational Drug Pharmacy. Once results come back, we have statisticians who work under the P.I. to analyze the data.

At the start of the study and throughout its duration, an internal research compliance department audits the study in full to ensure compliance with all regulations.

Once all this collaboration has happened and the results obtained, the P.I. puts everything together and presents and publishes the findings.

The Emerging Data on Vitamin D and COVID-19

In June of 2020, Gareth Davies, Attila Garami, and Joanna Byers published a preprint for a study that was intended to examine the relationship between COVID-19 severity and latitude. They'd noticed that the pandemic seemed to most severely affect locations in the northern hemisphere that overlapped with a pattern of seasonal vitamin D deficiency. They hypothesized that vitamin D status could play a causal role in COVID outcomes.

What is "causal inference"?

Causal inference (C.I.) rose out of artificial intelligence research and was brought into health research around 2000. Utilizing statistics that define causation mathematically, it can determine if causation can be inferred from observational data. The size of causal effect can also be calculated using C.I.

This is valuable because correlation of data alone does not necessarily determine causation. Correlation means that there is a relationship between two things, while causation refers to one thing causing another. This is an important aspect to note in research studies, because not all relationships that seem correlated, or tied together in some way, are actually causal relationships. Correlation does not prove causation. And establishing causation is what allows us to apply research in the best way possible.

How is correlation different from causation ?

Finding correlations can be the first step in finding a causal role, and correlations are important for that reason. This is true whether the two elements are directly related (both are increasing) or inversely related (one increases as the other decreases). However a correlation proves nothing: researchers must go beyond the correlation to find and document a causal role.

As an example, statistically significant, beautiful correlations have been discovered that make no sense at all, such as the nearly perfect direct correlation (98.5 percent) between the total revenue generated by arcades and the number of computer science doctorates awarded in the U.S. between the years 2000 to 2009.[21]

Did the arcade revenue contribute to those students achieving their degrees? You can probably think of a humorous reason why it might. However, investigating this correlation might find that revenues increased during that time because of a decrease in the cost of video games or an increase in sales of popular snacks and had nothing to do with how much money bored computer science students spent at the arcades.

---

21. Vigen, Tyler. *Spurious Correlations* (Hachette Books, 2015).

Because seasons are determined by latitude and winter offers a better environment for viral transmission, it wasn't surprising that transmission rates varied by latitude. Yet data also suggested that, beyond transmission, COVID-19 fatality rates (CFRs) were determined by latitude too. So not only was COVID being transmitted more frequently in certain latitudes, but people were also getting more severe cases. *This* was the surprising factor that prompted the authors of the study to explore what was going on.

They were drawn to explore vitamin D in relation to latitude because—since vitamin D is produced in the skin by sunlight—its deficiency is latitude- and season-dependent. During winter in locations outside the tropics, the UV Index (UVI) doesn't reach sufficient levels for the skin to produce vitamin D. The difference of UVI over seasons and latitude is known to correlate with and cause seasonal variations in serum levels of vitamin D.

Researchers were also aware of vitamin D's significant impact in the body, as vitamin D deficiency is associated with increased risk for cardiovascular diseases, infectious diseases, many cancers, dementia, type 2 diabetes, and more.

The researchers also considered Italy. It was one of the hardest-hit countries in Europe, and the country has some of the highest rates of vitamin D deficiency, also known as hypovitaminosis D. Seventy-six percent of women in Italy between ages 60 and 80 were found to have 25(OH)D levels below 12 ng/ml, the marker of deficiency.

What is 25(OH)D?

Researchers use a test called the 25-hydroxy vitamin D test, or 25(OH)D, as the best available marker to inform us about vitamin D status. Because 25(OH)D is the major form of vitamin D found circulating in the blood, it is considered a reliable indicator of the body's vitamin D supply. A low 25(OH)D result is a marker for a suboptimal vitamin D status.

The research team analyzed global daily reports of fatalities and recoveries from 239 locations between January 22, 2020 and April 9, 2020, drawing upon 1.6 million confirmed infections and covering a population of around one billion. The size and scope of the available data for the study was unprecedented.

By studying COVID-19 severity by latitude and season and then applying a causal inference framework, they sought to answer the question "Has vitamin D played a causal role in outbreak severity?"

They observed the following:

- In general, severe outbreaks with high fatality rates happened only in the northern hemisphere post-winter locations.
- In general, outbreaks in tropical and southern post-summer locations were mild.
- Northern outliers Canada, Germany, Japan, and South Korea all correlated with known low prevalence

of hypovitaminosis D (that is, where vitamin D deficiency rate is much lower) relative to countries with severe outbreaks, presumed to be due to either diets containing high amounts of fish or supplementation. (Actual cause is immaterial.)

- Southern outliers the Philippines, Indonesia, and Brazil, with unusually high case fatality rates, corresponded with evidence of high prevalence of hypovitaminosis D in at-risk populations.

- Pregnancy and infancy are typically high-risk groups for most diseases, yet in developed countries where these groups are routinely supplemented with vitamin D, they have curiously not shown up as high risk.

- Statistics for communities with genetically dark skin in the U.K. and U.S. have confirmed case fatality rates twice the average rate.[22] People with dark skin are known to produce less vitamin D through the interaction of sunlight with their skin and are more likely to be deficient.

Within the study, researchers also looked at historical evidence around vitamin D and earlier pandemics and epidemics. They noted that between 1930 and 1950, vitamin D supplementation was commonplace and vitamin D

---

22. Davies, Gareth, Attila R. Garami, and Joanna Byers. "Evidence Supports a Causal Role for Vitamin D Status in Global COVID-19 Outcomes," *medRxiv* (Preprint), June 9, 2020: https://www.medrxiv.org/content/10.1101/2020.05.0 1.20087965v3

deficiency was eradicated. Then in 1950, the practice was banned since uncontrolled dosing had led to hypercalcemia, and vitamin D deficiency then returned. When sunblocks with UVB blockers were introduced in the 1970s, it made the prevalence of deficiency worse.

Davies, Garami, and Byers wrote, "We note with interest that on the timeline of major influenza epidemics there is a 37-year period from 1920 to 1957 where no new flu strains seem to appear and no new pandemics occurred. This coincides with the only known period during which the population at large was routinely supplemented with vitamin D. This historical observation in alignment with our analysis verifies the causal role of vitamin D supplementation in respiratory disease pandemic prevention."[23]

The authors also pointed to several corroborating observational studies that appeared in preprint that showed a significant correlation between vitamin D deficiency in study subjects and the severity of their COVID outcomes. They wrote that while none of these observational studies served as proof of causation, they did show significant correlations between vitamin D and COVID severity that fully aligned with the authors' study results.

Davies, Garami, and Byers concluded by stating: "Based on the evidence from our causal inference analysis, we strongly recommend vitamin D supplementation to ensure

---

23. Ibid.

sufficiency across the global population . . . Vitamin D prophylaxis can be implemented immediately in advance of vaccines and medications under development, and moreover, offers long-term added value for the general health status of the population . . . Ensuring population-wide vitamin D sufficiency could mitigate seasonal respiratory epidemics, decrease our dependence on pharmaceutical solutions, reduce hospitalizations, and thus greatly lower healthcare costs while significantly increasing quality of life."[24]

This was a revealing study around vitamin D as it related to COVID-19, one that offered a wide context for how Vitamin D might fit into the puzzle. Further studies continue to suggest vitamin D is important.

A meta-analysis on the relationship between vitamin D deficiency and COVID-19 severity was published in October of 2020. This meta-analysis included 8,176 COVID patients participating in 56 studies. The mean age was 58 years old. Researchers asked, "What is the prevalence of vitamin D deficiency in people with COVID-19? Is vitamin D deficiency associated with COVID-19 severity?"

Across 17 studies, they found vitamin D deficiency in 39 percent of the individuals with COVID-19. They also observed that individuals with severe COVID-19 exhibited 65

24. Davies, Gareth, Attila R. Garami, and Joanna Byers. "Evidence Supports a Causal Role for Vitamin D Status in Global COVID-19 Outcomes," *medRxiv* (Preprint), June 9, 2020: https://www.medrxiv.org/content/10.1101/2020.05.0 1.20087965v3

percent more vitamin D deficiency compared with mild cases of the disease. The authors stated that vitamin D deficiency correlated with COVID severity, especially in the elderly, and that deficiency was related to the progression of COVID-19 and to mortality. They're careful to note that other factors like comorbidities in patients must be considered.[25]

Other studies also showed a relationship between vitamin D and COVID. Based on the strength of emerging data, 210 scientists from around the world gathered together to call on governments, public health officials, doctors, and healthcare workers worldwide to undertake efforts to increase vitamin D levels in the adult population. In their joint letter, they wrote the following:

> Research shows low vitamin D levels appear to promote COVID-19 infections, and related hospitalizations and deaths. Given its safety, *we call for immediate widespread increased vitamin D intakes.*
>
> Vitamin D modulates thousands of genes and many aspects of immune function, both innate and adaptive. The scientific evidence shows that:
>
> - Higher vitamin D blood levels are associated with lower rates of SARS-CoV-2 infection.

25. Pereira, Marcos, Alialdo Dantas Damascena, Laylla Mirella Galvão Azevedo, Tarcio de Almeida Oliveira, and Jerusa da Mota Santana. "Vitamin D Deficiency Aggravates COVID-19: Systematic Review and Meta-Analysis," *Critical Reviews in Food Science and Nutrition*, November 4, 2020: 1-9. https://doi.org/10.1080/1 0408398.2020.1841090; https://pubmed.ncbi.nlm.nih.gov/33146028/

- Higher vitamin D levels are associated with lower risk of a severe case (hospitalization, ICU, or death).

- Some intervention studies (including RCTs [randomized controlled trials]) indicate that vitamin D can be a very effective treatment.

- Many papers reveal several biological mechanisms by which vitamin D influences COVID-19.

- Causal inference modeling, Hill's criteria, the intervention studies, and the biological mechanisms indicate that vitamin D's influence on COVID-19 is very likely causal, not just correlation.

Vitamin D is well known to be essential, but most people do not get enough. Two common definitions of inadequacy are deficiency <20ng/ml (50nmol/L), the target of most governmental organizations, and insufficiency <30ng/ml (75nmol/L), the target of several medical societies and experts.

Too many people have levels below these targets. **Rates of vitamin D deficiency, <20ng/ml, exceed 33 percent of the population in most of the world. Most estimates of insufficiency <30ng/ml are well over 50 percent (but much higher in many countries).** Rates are even higher in winter, and several groups have notably worse deficiency: the overweight, those with dark skin (especially far from the equator), and care home residents. These same groups face increased COVID-19 risk . . .

Evidence to date suggests the possibility that the COVID-19 pandemic sustains itself in large part through infection of those with low vitamin D, and that deaths are concentrated largely in those with deficiency. The mere possibility that this is so should compel urgent gathering of more vitamin D data. Even without more data, **the preponderance of evidence indicates that increased vitamin D would help reduce infections, hospitalizations, ICU admissions, and deaths.**[26]

The signatories closed their letter with a plea, "Please act immediately."[27]

I agree that the research suggests enough benefit of vitamin D supplementation that we need to act on it.

Initially, we couldn't be sure if the reasons for the prevalence of vitamin D deficiency in patients with poor COVID outcomes was because the vitamin D deficiency itself contributed to their outcome, or because vitamin D deficiency tended to be present in patients who were more susceptible for other reasons (such as having comorbidities). More research is still needed, but it's looking more and more like vitamin D is a significant factor independent of any other.

---

26. "Over 200 Scientists & Doctors Call for Increase Vitamin D Use to Combat COVID-19," VitaminDforAll.org, December 7, 2020: https://vitamindforall. org/letter.html

27. Ibid.

My most recent research is beginning to bear this out as well. In a study we did in Cleveland, after accounting for age, gender, race, comorbidities, and body mass index (BMI), only two factors remained independently associated with more severe COVID-19 illness: vitamins D and K2 deficiency.

Vitamin D seems to be a critical piece of this COVID-19 and immunity puzzle.

There has been some growing recognition of this, yet there's another important consideration that public discussion around vitamin D hasn't yet emphasized. This research around vitamin D needs to be considered alongside other research—research around vitamin K2.

CHAPTER 5

The Critical Impact of Vitamin K2

Further studies are suggesting that as powerful as vitamin D is, we should do more than simply consider it on its own. We've learned about a missing link that has hardly touched public awareness and is new in the research community, by and large. Recent studies suggest it may be a major piece of this COVID-19 and immunity puzzle: vitamin K2. Our own COVID research is suggesting vitamin K2 has a significant effect on its own in alleviating the severity of COVID, in addition to its beneficial effect in conjunction with vitamin D.

Before we explore that further, I'd like to take a step back from COVID-19 to establish a broader context for vitamin K2, as we did with vitamin D. This is especially important because vitamin K2 is a micronutrient most people rarely think about.

I was recently speaking with a friend (a nurse) about vitamins D and K2. She'd heard about the general benefits of vitamin D years ago and had a feeling she should probably be taking it as a supplement, because a test had indicated her blood levels were low. She hadn't considered it serious enough to take action. Then she added, "I really have no idea what K2 does. I never hear about it or consider it at all."

This tends to be true for most of the population. Even doctors rarely think about—or understand—K2.

Vitamin K was discovered in 1929 by the Danish scientist Henrik Dam. While investigating the role of dietary cholesterol by feeding chickens a diet without fat, he and his colleagues discovered the chickens were experiencing frequent bleeding. When they added cholesterol back into the diet, the bleeding continued, so Dam hypothesized that another compound missing from the diet was responsible. Eventually, through studying hempseed, he discovered a factor that prevented bleeding. It was referenced in a German journal as "Koagulations vitamin," which then became known as vitamin K.[28] Soon after, American biochemist Edward Doisy determined the chemical structure of vitamin K and synthesized it for the first time. Dam and Doisy received the Nobel Prize in Medicine in 1943 for their work discovering the vitamin, a family of K forms which later became known as K1. These K1 forms are also known as phylloquinones.

In the 1950s, a group of various K forms was recognized that were different from what Dam and Doisy had discov-

28. Mandal, Ananya. "Vitamin K Biochemistry," *News Medical Life Sciences*, updated April 24, 2019: https://www.news-medical.net/health/Vitamin-K-Biochemistry.aspx

ered; this group was designated as K2. The forms within this group are also known as menaquinones.

What do the numbers mean?

The different menaquinone forms of vitamin K2 differ in the length of the carbon side chain they contain, and are named by the number of five-carbon building block units called isoprene making up that side chain. They are designated as menaquinone-n (or MK-n), where n is the number of building block units in the side chain. Many researchers have selected the MK-7 or MK-4 forms of vitamin K2 for study, and supplements bear this designation as well, with MK-7 being the preferred, most stable, and most effective version.

While K1 is a hepatic form, stored in the liver and mostly known to affect blood coagulation, K2 is extrahepatic, which means it is found outside the liver. It has been found in many body tissues, and it has an entirely different function in the body. Yet the association with the Nobel Prize-winning "Koagulations vitamin" remains. Even today, most people who know something about vitamin K1 and its role in coagulation assume vitamin K2 plays a similar, limited role. The two distinct vitamins have been indistinguishable in people's minds for decades—lumped together as simply "vitamin K" even by some dietary authorities—and the time has come to uncouple them.

Do the studies refer to vitamin K1 or K2?

Some studies don't specify whether they are talking about vitamin K1 or K2. An important part of any scientific study is determining what will be measured and what those measurements mean for the conclusions. No reliable methods for measuring Vitamin K1 and K2 directly in the blood have been developed—unlike vitamin D, which can be measured directly using the 25(OH)D test. While there are ways to identify which form was involved indirectly (through measurement of what's called K-dependent proteins), some studies don't identify the form of the vitamin being discussed. It's important not to assume it's K1 or K2 if that isn't stated. So if the study didn't identify the form beyond "vitamin K" with no number, it's reported here in the same way. Possible modes of recycling of vitamin K1 and of converting between K1 and K2 are under investigation.

Molecular Structures of Vitamin K1 and Two K2 Variants

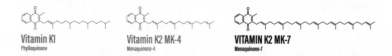

The molecular structure of vitamin K1 and two of the vitamin K2 variations.

Vitamin K2 has been neglected for a long time.

Some interesting explorations concerning vitamin K2 happened quietly even before vitamin K2 was officially identified in the 50s. Around the time that Dam and Doisy were exploring K1, Dr. Weston Price was exploring traditional diets in an attempt to uncover what aspects of nutrition may influence tooth decay.

After studying groups of Inuit, Pacific Islanders, Australian Aborigines, New Zealand Maori, Swiss Highlanders, and South American Indians, he observed that those raised on indigenous diets had healthier teeth compared to those eating modern diets. He realized there must be some nutrient they consumed that made the difference. In continuing his work, he discovered a fat-soluble vitamin he called "Activator X," which seemed to have a significant effect on bones and teeth and was often missing in the modern diet. Activator X is now believed to be vitamin K2.

And Dr. Price seemed to be right: while vitamin K2 is present in some traditional diets and diets of the past (like those of samurai warriors who consumed large amounts of a fermented soybean dish called natto), it's noticeably absent in most modern diets.

Yet we're learning it is crucial to the body.

The Recognized Benefits of Vitamin K2

Until recently, the primary benefits of vitamin K2 have been assumed to be associated with bone and cardiovascular health. It's true that vitamin K2 has powerful impacts in these areas. In fact, it's an essential vitamin necessary for both bones and the heart because it regulates the transport and distribution of calcium in the body. Calcium is a building block for bones and teeth, and it plays other roles. It can also be deposited in places where it can do damage, when it is in excess. As part of its journey to reach the bones and teeth, calcium first must cross into the bloodstream—an essential step. Yet if an excess of calcium reaches the bloodstream and isn't properly funneled into the bones, it can lead to calcification of arteries, reducing elasticity of blood vessels and increasing the risk of cardiovascular events.

Progression of Atherosclerosis

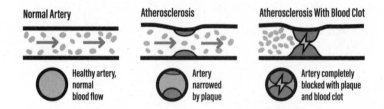

An example of how calcification of blood vessels reduces blood flow and can be completely blocked by a blood clot.

That's where vitamin K2 comes in, in concert with vitamin D.

To direct calcium to the bones and away from the arteries, vitamin K2 activates two key proteins, osteocalcin and matrix Gla-protein (MGP), through a chemical reaction called carboxylation. As we've touched on earlier, osteocalcin helps integrate calcium into the bones. MGP binds calcium that remains in the bloodstream, to prevent buildup in the arteries. With these functions, vitamin K2 is absolutely fundamental to bone and heart health. A collection of studies looking at the effects of vitamin K2 supplementation on deficiency underscore the vitamin's importance here.

In a double-blind, randomized, placebo-controlled study of 244 healthy postmenopausal women, participants were given either a daily dose of 180 mcg K2 as MK-7 or a placebo over a period of three years. The study found that long-term supplementation of vitamin K2 as MK-7 significantly decreased age-related decline in bone mineral density (BMD) and bone mineral content (BMC) at the lumbar spine and femoral neck. It also reduced the loss of vertebral height of the lower thoracic region at the mid-site of the vertebrae.

Additionally, supplementation also significantly increased serum levels of active/carboxylated osteocalcin and lowered the levels of inactive/uncarboxylated osteocalcin. Higher levels of carboxylated osteocalcin, the active form, have been associated with lower BMD and greater fracture risk. These findings suggest vitamin K2 MK-7 supplementation at the right dose may help prevent age-related bone loss in postmenopausal women.[29]

---

29. Knapen, M.H., N.E. Drummen, E. Smit, C. Vermeer, and E. Theuwissen. "Three-Year Low-Dose Menaquinone-7 Supplementation Helps Decrease Bone Loss in Healthy Post-Menopausal Women," *Osteoporosis International,* 2013, 24(9): 2499–507. https://pubmed.ncbi.nlm.nih.gov/23525894/

In summary: vitamin K2 MK-7 was shown to slow bone loss

This high quality study showed over a three-year timeframe that vitamin K2, as the MK-7 form supplement in a higher daily dose (180 mcg, 180 micrograms), significantly slowed loss of bone and related damage to the spine in postmenopausal women. The study also related those effects to an increased level of osteocalcin, measured in the blood in its active, carboxylated form. These results show a causal relationship that supports the recommendation to supplement vitamin K2 MK-7 at higher dosages than are often recommended. No side effects of the higher dosage were observed.

Another study explored whether the intake of vitamin K1 or K2 through dietary sources was related to aortic calcification and coronary heart disease. The study followed 4,807 participants for seven to ten years and monitored their health in three areas: incidents of coronary heart disease (CHD), all-cause mortality (all causes of mortality), and aortic atherosclerosis, along with correlations to vitamin K1 and K2 intake. While they found no consistent correlations between vitamin K1 intake and CHD, all-cause mortality, or aortic atherosclerosis, the results for vitamin K2 were striking. Researchers discovered a strong inverse relationship between vitamin K2 intake and severe arterial calcification. They also found significant inverse correlations between vitamin K2 intake and incidents of CHD, CHD mortality, and all causes of mortality.[30]

30. Geleijnse, J.M., Cees Vermeer, Diederick E. Grobbee, Leon J. Schurgers, Marjo H.J. Knapen, Irene M. van der Meer, Albert Hofman, and Jacqueline

> **In summary: dietary intake of vitamin K2 was inversely correlated with heart disease, death from heart disease, and all causes of death**
>
> The 4,807-participant study by Geleijnse et al. (2004) clearly showed that increased vitamin K2 intake reduced the incidence of heart disease and atherosclerosis as well as all causes of death. Vitamin K1 intake did not show these correlations, demonstrating clearly that the roles of vitamin K1 and K2 are very different.

Recent research by many groups is reinforcing the value of vitamin K2 in bone and heart health and what a vital substance it is for our bodies. As an infectious disease specialist, the new frontier emerging around vitamin K2 as it relates to COVID-19 is even more exciting to me. As results come in, my passion around it is growing.

So now let's look at how the initial connection between vitamin K2 and COVID-19 was made.

Vitamin K2's Effect on Inflammation

Inflammation is at the forefront of all disease.

HIV, for example, is a state of chronic inflammation—not the kind of inflammation that causes stiff joints, but systemic

---

C.M. Witteman. "Dietary Intake of Menaquinone Is Associated with a Reduced Risk of Coronary Heart Disease: The Rotterdam Study," *Journal of Nutrition*, 2004, 134(11): 3100–5. https://pubmed.ncbi.nlm.nih.gov/15514282/

inflammation throughout the body. When you check markers of inflammation in HIV patients' blood, they're very elevated compared to healthy control patients the same age. Even if people have been on HIV medications for years and their HIV is well controlled, their inflammation continues to be very high.

I've conducted studies linking HIV patients' inflammation to the onset of diabetes, cardiovascular disease, and bone disease. There are also studies in the general population linking inflammation to heart disease and even cancer.

From all of these and especially from the HIV studies, we have a growing conviction that inflammation drives many comorbidities.

Among other reasons, I'm excited to be researching vitamin K2 because of its likely effect on inflammation. Studies suggest that vitamin K2 plays a role in downregulation of NF-kB, which can stop a whole cascade of downstream inflammation. By blocking inflammation, vitamin K2 may be able to help the general population and significantly help people who have conditions known to involve a high level of chronic inflammation, such as rheumatoid arthritis, lupus, and HIV.

Other Effects of K2

Vitamin K2 is turning out to be a hidden wonder in a variety of interesting ways. One of these is its effect on maximal cardiac output, the amount of blood the heart pumps through the circulatory system in a minute.

Following eight weeks of vitamin K2 MK-7 supplementation, trained athletes indicated a 12 percent increase in maximal cardiac output compared to trained athletes receiving a placebo. Researchers estimate this provided results equivalent to six to nine months of continuous training. While this isn't clearly related to immunity, it points to the range of possibility we're discovering with K2.[31]

31. McFarlin, B.K., A.L. Henning, and A.S. Venable. "Oral Consumption of Vitamin K2 for 8 Weeks Associated With Increased Maximal Cardiac Output During Exercise," *Altern. Ther. Health Med.*, 2017, 23(4): 26-32. https://pubmed.ncbi.nlm.nih.gov/28646812/

The Emerging Data on Vitamin K and COVID-19

Soon after the pandemic began, Dr. Rob Janssen was asked by Dr. Anton Dofferhoff to join a group studying biomarkers in COVID-19.

Who are the people behind the work?

Rob Janssen, M.D., is a pulmonary specialist and translational lung researcher who was at Canisius Wilhelmina Hospital in Nijmegen, The Netherlands, at the time of this writing. His focus has been on elastic fiber metabolism in pulmonary fibrosis and emphysema.

Anton Dofferhoff, M.D., Ph.D., is with the Department of Internal Medicine, Canisius-Wilhelmina Hospital, Nijmegen, The Netherlands.

Janssen had previously been studying elastic fiber degradation in chronic obstructive pulmonary disease (COPD), looking first at vitamin D and, more recently, at vitamin K. In his work with vitamin K2 and COPD, he had observed an inverse relationship with elastic fiber degradation: the lower the levels of vitamin K2, the higher the elastic fiber degradation. He had also noted that in COPD and lung fibrosis patients, vitamin K and the amino acid desmosine levels were always correlated.

So when Janssen began studying biomarkers in COVID-19, the first thing he looked at was desmosine. When he found high levels of desmosine in the blood of COVID patients, he knew they should look at their vitamin K2 levels. Janssen and his colleagues became some of the first researchers to study the relationship between vitamin K2 and COVID. They hypothesized that vitamin K status was reduced in patients with severe COVID-19.

What is desmosine?

Desmosine is an amino acid found only in elastin, a protein found in connective tissues of the skin, lungs, and arteries. Detecting desmosine as a breakdown product in bodily fluids indicates elastin degradation, which is associated with disease.

To assess vitamin K2 status, they measured the blood concentration of desphospho-uncarboxylated matrix Gla protein (dp-ucMGP). This is the inactive form of a vitamin K-dependent protein, and its concentration is inversely related to vitamin K status. In other words, high levels of dp-ucMGP equate to suboptimal vitamin K2 status. They also measured desmosine, which indicates rates of elastin degradation.

They discovered that dp-ucMGP levels were significantly elevated in COVID-19 patients compared to control patients, which means that COVID patients had lower levels of vitamin K. They also found that higher dp-ucMGP levels and desmosine levels were significantly associated with severe COVID cases.

In conclusion, they wrote: "Vitamin K status was reduced in patients with COVID-19 and related to poor prognosis. Also, low vitamin K status seems to be associated with accelerated elastin degradation. An intervention trial is now needed to assess whether vitamin K administration improves outcomes in patients with COVID-19."[32]

32. Dofferhoff, Anton S.M., et al. "Reduced Vitamin K Status as a Potentially Modifiable Risk Factor of Severe Coronavirus Disease 2019," *Clinical Infectious*

The First Link Between Vitamin K and COVID-19

When Dr. Janssen discovered a link between vitamin K and COVID-19, he was excited. As a researcher, he always sought to look for answers in a different direction than expected, and here he found something new and promising, something that could possibly help—and with no side effects.

The team received media attention over their findings in Europe, but attention to vitamin K quickly waned. Dr. Janssen notes that many people, including doctors, still have the wrong impression about vitamin K, thinking its benefits impact only coagulation. Many doctors are also surprised by the study findings; they expect the opposite. Dr. Janssen himself hadn't realized or expected vitamin K to have such an important role in blood vessels and be linked to the lungs. Now, as someone who has researched both vitamins D and K, he feels vitamin K might be the more promising of the two.

In 2021, Dr. Janssen continued his exploration of vitamin K with a new study looking at whether populations with less recycling of the vitamin have less chance of severe COVID-19. (Vitamin K activates proteins through a carboxylation reaction, which leaves it in a reduced state [lacking oxygen]; this inactive form of vitamin K can be recycled by re-oxidizing it with an enzyme, vitamin K epoxide reduc-

Diseases, August 27, 2020: https://academic.oup.com/cid/advance-article/doi/10.1093/cid/ciaa1258/5898121

tase.) In addition, Janssen began work on a vitamin K intervention trial in COVID-19 patients.

Janssen's work was the first connection made between vitamin K and COVID-19, and it sparked new possibilities and inspired further studies.

Research led by Allan Linneberg has continued to explore the link between COVID-19 and vitamin K. Linneberg and his team wanted to reproduce Janssen's study to see if they could confirm the results. As part of this, Linneberg's team sought to test the hypothesis that low vitamin K status was a common feature of hospitalized COVID patients compared to population controls, and furthermore, that low vitamin K status was a predictor of mortality in hospitalized COVID-19 patients.

This study also measured dp-ucMGP levels in a total of 138 hospitalized COVID patients. Thirty-six of these patients died within 30 days from joining the study, and 43 patients died within 90 days. Among the study patients, both 30-day and 90-day mortality outcomes were significantly associated with increased levels of dp-ucMGP. (Remember, high levels of dp-ucMGP indicate low levels of vitamin K.) Mortality rates here were also significantly associated with high age, hypertension, and cardiovascular disease.

The study authors wrote, "There is an urgent need for measures to improve the outcome and long-term consequences of COVID-19. Supplementation with vitamin K represents an inexpensive and simple-to-use intervention. It is of potential interest that obesity is a predictor of outcome of SARS-CoV-2 infection. This could be in line with our recent report that obesity was strongly associated with higher levels of dp-ucMGP (indicating low vitamin K status) providing a possible explanation for the link between obesity and COVID-19."[33]

Dr. Linneberg's journey with vitamin K

Dr. Linneberg first became interested in vitamin K research around 2010, through a collaborator who was interested in the vitamin. They tried to raise funding but didn't receive it, and so his work remained in other areas until recently, when he received a grant to study vitamin K and cardiovascular health. Soon after the pandemic began, he came across Janssen's study on COVID-19 and vitamin K. He found the results so intriguing he immediately began looking for collaborators to continue the research.

The study authors concluded by noting that vitamin K status was confirmed to be significantly lower in hospitalized COVID-19 patients compared to population controls and that low vitamin K status predicted mortality in COVID-19 patients. They also stated that randomized clinical trials

33. Linneberg, A., et al., "Low Vitamin K Status Predicts Mortality in a Cohort of 138 Hospitalized Patients with COVID-19," *medRxiv* (Preprint), December 23, 2020: https://www.medrxiv.org/content/10.1101/2020.12.21.20248613v1.full-text

were needed to determine if vitamin K supplementation in COVID-19 patients can change the course of the disease and prevent death or long-term consequences.[34] This is the next step for Linneberg and his team.

Who is Dr. Linneberg?

Allan Linneberg, M.D., Ph.D., serves as Clinical Professor of Integration of Epidemiological Methods in Clinical Research, University of Copenhagen, and as Director of the Center for Clinical Research and Disease Prevention, Bispebjerg and Frederiksberg Hospital, in Denmark. Dr. Linneberg and his team were able to confirm the research results of Dr. Rob Janssen on correlating vitamin K insufficiency in patients with COVID-19 and the inverse correlation between extra-hepatic vitamin K status and elastic fiber degradation.

As we learn more about the SARS-CoV-2 virus and how it attacks the human body, we are learning more about how the immune system works and how we may be able to help the body fight the virus. A recent discovery was reported in a *Science* journal article about a new type of binding site found in three places on the SARS-CoV-2 spike protein. The spike protein has been shown as a primary enabler for viral entry into human cells.[35] Those spike protein binding sites are

---

34. Ibid.

35. Toelzer, C., K. Gupta, S.K.N. Yadav, U. Borucu, A.D. Davidson, M. Kavanagh Williamson, D.K. Shoemark, F. Garzoni, O. Staufer, R. Milligan, J. Capin, A.J.

specific for fatty acid (FA) residues such as the essential FA linoleic acid. When these three sites are occupied by FAs or related molecules, the spike protein's structure changes to a "locked" conformation that is unable to interact with ACE2 binding domains and may reduce infectivity. Only in the unlocked, "open" form with nothing occupying those binding sites can the virus infect cells. In a computational molecular dynamics (MD) simulation study, the same researchers further explored other structurally similar molecules that bind effectively ("dock") with those fatty acid binding sites. They found that vitamin K2 bound more strongly than other molecules tested, including a library of FDA-approved drugs like dexamethasone (a steroid that has been shown to improve outcomes for severely ill COVID-19 patients) plus nutrients such as vitamin D, vitamin A, and cholesterol.[36] The results of this study suggest that further research on vitamin K2's potential ability to reduce the infectivity of the SARS-CoV-2 spike protein is warranted.

Mulholland, J. Spatz, D. Fitzgerald, I. Berger, and C. Schaffitzel. "Free fatty acid binding pocket in the locked structure of SARS-CoV-2 spike protein," *Science*, 2020, 370: 725-730. https://science.sciencemag.org/content/370/6517/725

36. Shoemark, D.K., C.K. Colenso, C. Toelzer, K. Gupta, R.B. Sessions A.D. Davidson, I. Berger, C. Schaffitzel, J. Spencer, and A.J. Mulholland. "Molecular Simulations Suggest Vitamins, Retinoids and Steroids as Ligands of the Free Fatty Acid Pocket of the SARS-CoV-2 Spike Protein," *Angewandte Chemie International Edition*, 2021, 60: 2014. https://onlinelibrary.wiley.com/doi/10.1002/anie.202015639

Vitamin K2 MK-7

Some studies around vitamin K2 refer to one specific mena-quinone: menaquinone 7, which is also called MK-7 or K2 MK-7. Why this particular form?

Well, it seems to be the most powerful.

First, vitamin K2 MK-7 exhibits the most bioavailability, which means a greater portion of the vitamin enters the circulation and is able to have an effect. It also has the longest half-life (the amount of time it takes for half of the original concentration to be degraded) of all the K vitamins: the half-life of K2 MK-7 is 72 hours while the half-life of K2 MK-4, for example, is two hours. This means it remains available in the body for longer. Intestinal absorption rates of various MK forms are also different, which influences how effective they are at activating K-dependent proteins like osteocalcin and matrix Gla-protein. MK-7 is more efficiently absorbed than other forms.

For these reasons, MK-7 is generally regarded as the best form for use in vitamin K2 supplements. Moreover, K2 MK-7 is the only form with European Food Safety Authority approval.

The studies I've just discussed are admittedly heavy on technical terms, but I share them in detail because they're compelling. They truly are the beginning of a new frontier of research. Inspired by these initial findings around vitamin K2, a handful of other researchers are now exploring vitamin K2 as it relates to COVID-19, including myself.

How Dietary Deficiencies of Vitamins D and K2 Affect Inflammation in the Body and the Immune System

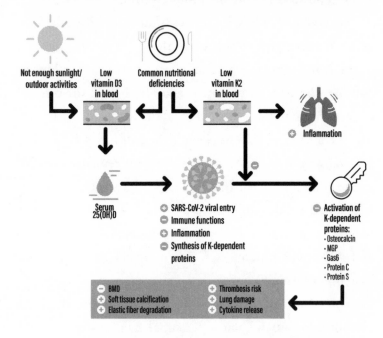

Dietary intake of vitamins D and K2 without supplementation can lead to combined deficiency and a host of poor health outcomes. Adapted from Goddek, 2020.[37]

37. Goddek, Simon. "Vitamin D3 and K2 and Their Potential Contribution to Reducing the COVID-19 Mortality Rate," *International Journal of Infectious Diseases*, October 1, 2020, 99: 286–90. https://doi.org/10.1016/j.ijid.2020.07.080

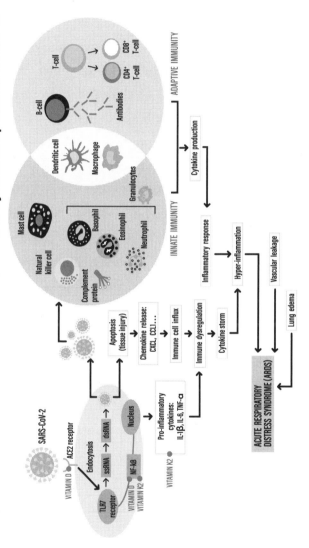

Vitamins D and K2 support the immune system's response to COVID-19 in many ways. Vitamin K2's roles affect the "cytokine storm" in the fourth stage.

At the start of the pandemic, my team began putting together a central biorepository of samples from COVID-19 patients, collecting every type of sample we could—stool, urine, blood, saliva, sputum, tracheal secretion. By January of 2021, we had collected around 18,000 samples and had gathered a significant amount of clinical data from them. The biorepository has been a way for researchers to get samples quickly without having to first enroll new patients in a study, a process that can sometimes take up to a year. Now, researchers have immediate access to samples that are helping them ask and answer important questions about COVID-19.

My team and I recently performed a study investigating vitamin K2 using these samples. Since all the earlier data were on the sickest (hospitalized) patients, we wanted to study a wider variety of clinical presentations. We included patients who tested positive but were asymptomatic as well as patients who had mild cases, moderate cases, and severe cases requiring hospitalization or that resulted in death. Then we examined various biomarkers in their samples, such as age, sex, race, BMI, comorbidities, vitamin D status, and vitamin K status.

Our first data set confirmed our hypothesis that both poor vitamin K2 and vitamin D status significantly predicted worse illness.

We discovered that vitamin K2 and vitamin D insufficiencies were the most significant independent risk factors for the severity of COVID-19, after adjusting for all other factors.

Adjusting to look at factors independently is very important. Let's look at race for an example of why this is important. It is now well known that black race is associated with a worse outcome after COVID-19 infection, but to date, we do not know why. Is it due to more comorbidities, or late access to care? Another explanation would be low vitamin D, as people of color make less vitamin D and are highly prone to vitamin D deficiency. Similar observations could explain why BMI has been associated with more COVID cases and with worse outcomes. High BMI is a risk factor for vitamin D deficiency. So if you have obesity (high BMI) with the associated vitamin D deficiency, you may have a worse COVID-19 outcome. This is why in our study we adjusted for BMI, race, and other factors. In doing so, we found that vitamin D and K deficiencies were the best predictors of COVID-19 disease outcome.

For every doubling of uncarboxylated GMP (which is a sign of vitamin K2 insufficiency), there was a doubling of risk for COVID-19 severity. This shows how closely tied together COVID-19 outcomes and K status are.

My team's research data is still coming in, but preliminary results are already exciting. I know we're discovering something people need to know, something that can possibly keep them out of the hospital and away from a poor COVID outcome. (That is, if people take a preventative approach and get their vitamin levels in good shape *before* getting COVID. It's not yet known if taking vitamin K2 supplements after you are infected with COVID-19 will be a benefit in fighting the disease.)

As exciting as vitamin K2 is on its own, I'd now like to turn to the most valuable way to consider the vitamin—paired with vitamin D. While it's important to understand both of these essential micronutrients as they function individually, they have a truly synergistic partnership. Let's take a look.

CHAPTER 6

The Powerful Synergy of Vitamins D and K2

To understand the close synergy of vitamins D and K2, it's helpful to first return to a broader look at their function in the immune system as COVID-19 progresses.

During the immune response to an infection, vitamin D is needed to downregulate the expression of ACE2 receptors. This gives the virus less opportunity to enter cells. Vitamins D and K2 are both used throughout the immune response to downregulate NF-kB signaling and the secretion of cytokines. If NF-kB signaling and cytokine secretion are not downregulated, they can lead to the dangerous cytokine storm. Vitamin K2 is used in preventing thrombosis and vascular damage, which can be serious issues as COVID progresses.

This helps to illustrate how, in COVID-19, vitamins D and K2 affect the immune response in various ways and at various times. Both are necessary for a healthy immune response as the disease moves through the body.

Specific Roles of Vitamins D and K2 in the Body's Immune Response to COVID-19

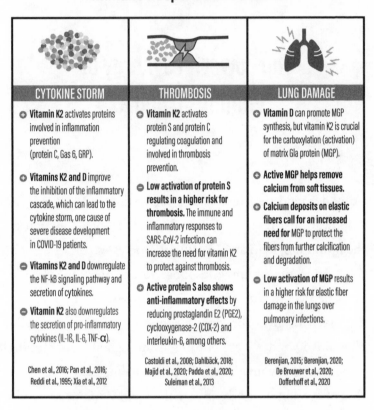

CYTOKINE STORM	THROMBOSIS	LUNG DAMAGE
⊕ **Vitamin K2** activates proteins involved in inflammation prevention (protein C, Gas 6, GRP).	⊕ **Vitamin K2** activates protein S and protein C regulating coagulation and involved in thrombosis prevention.	⊕ **Vitamin D** can promote MGP synthesis, but vitamin K2 is crucial for the carboxylation (activation) of matrix Gla protein (MGP).
⊕ **Vitamins K2 and D** improve the inhibition of the inflammatory cascade, which can lead to the cytokine storm, one cause of severe disease development in COVID-19 patients.	⊖ **Low activation of protein S results in a higher risk for thrombosis.** The immune and inflammatory responses to SARS-CoV-2 infection can increase the need for vitamin K2 to protect against thrombosis.	⊕ **Active MGP helps remove calcium from soft tissues.**
⊖ **Vitamins K2 and D** downregulate the NF-kB signaling pathway and secretion of cytokines.		⊕ **Calcium deposits on elastic fibers call for an increased need for** MGP to protect the fibers from further calcification and degradation.
⊖ **Vitamin K2** also downregulates the secretion of pro-inflammatory cytokines (IL-1ß, IL-6, TNF-α).	⊕ **Active protein S also shows anti-inflammatory effects** by reducing prostaglandin E2 (PGE2), cyclooxygenase-2 (COX-2) and interleukin-6, among others.	⊖ **Low activation of MGP** results in a higher risk for elastic fiber damage in the lungs over pulmonary infections.
Chen et al., 2016; Pan et al., 2016; Reddi et al., 1995; Xia et al., 2012	Castoldi et al., 2008; Dahlbäck, 2018; Majid et al., 2020; Padda et al., 2020; Suleiman et al., 2013	Berenjian, 2015; Berenjian, 2020; De Brouwer et al., 2020; Dofferhoff et al., 2020

Vitamins D and K2 are involved in many functions, including signaling in the immune system, and have been shown to prevent the cytokine storm that can happen during stage four of the COVID-19 disease.

We also can understand the synergy of these two vitamins by looking at their role in bone health. Vitamin D increases the expression of osteocalcin and matrix Gla protein (MGP), but these proteins remain inactive without vitamin K2.

A Japanese clinical trial looked at the effect of taking vitamin D3 with K2 in postmenopausal women with osteoporosis who had a similar pre-trial bone mineral density (BMD). The subjects were randomized to take either calcium alone, D3 alone, K2 alone, or a combination of D3 and K2. Subjects who took only calcium showed a significantly decreased BMD compared to those subjects taking either D3 alone or K2 alone, who showed significantly higher levels of BMD. The greatest increase in BMD, though, was reported in the group given the combination of vitamin D3 and K2.[38]

Vitamins D and K2 are meant to work together.

Vitamins D and K2 not only work together synergistically, vitamin K2 also protects the body against too much vitamin D. By only focusing on one you don't receive the full benefit the two vitamins can offer together. The benefits go beyond simply benefitting from both vitamins' complementary roles.

First, having a combined deficiency of both vitamin D and vitamin K may amplify mortality risks. A 2020 study[39]

38. Iwamoto, J., Takeda, T., and Ichimura, S. "Effect of combined administration of vitamin D3 and vitamin K2 on bone mineral density of the lumbar spine in postmenopausal women with osteoporosis," *Journal of Orthopaedic Science*, 2020, 5(6): 546-551. https://pubmed.ncbi.nlm.nih.gov/11180916/

39. van Ballegooijen, Adriana J., Joline W.J. Beulens, Lyanne M. Kieneker, Martin H. de Borst, Ron T. Gansevoort, Ido P. Kema, Leon J. Schurgers, Marc G. Vervloet, and Stephan J.L. Bakker. "Combined Low Vitamin D and K Status

looking at a group of middle-aged men and women found a combined low vitamin D and K status in 20 percent of the participants. Looking at this group over a span of at least 14 years, researchers discovered that their combined low vitamin D and vitamin K status was associated with a greater risk of all-cause mortality (death from all combined causes) than the sum of the risks from low vitamin D status alone and low vitamin K status alone. In other words, if vitamin D deficiency is X risk and vitamin K deficiency is Y risk, the risk from having deficiencies of both is greater than $X+Y$. Their combined benefit was more than double the benefit of either vitamin by itself.

Second, part of the discussion around vitamin D is that too much of it, alone, can sometimes have detrimental effects, including unwanted calcification. That's one of the essential reasons it should be paired with K2. Vitamin K2 is healthy for the body on its own, but it is also essential as a companion to vitamin D because of its complementary role in calcium metabolism. This is a critical point.

Remember that vitamin D transports calcium through the gut wall into the bloodstream. Once in the bloodstream, calcium will eventually get to the bones. However, taking a lot of vitamin D (without also taking supportive levels of vitamin K2) can potentially lead to a surplus of calcium in the blood, which can lead to calcification of arteries.

Vitamin K2 prevents this because it activates the osteocalcin and MGP proteins needed to prevent the calcium buildup

Amplifies Mortality Risk: A Prospective Study," *European Journal of Nutrition*, August 17, 2020: https://doi.org/10.1007/s00394-020-02352-8

in arteries that can lead to calcification. (As a reminder, osteocalcin helps bring calcium from the bloodstream into the bones, and MGP binds calcium that remains in the blood.)

For this reason, we believe vitamin D must be considered together with vitamin K2.

The Need for Vitamin K2 With Vitamin D

Researcher Simon Goddek wrote of the need for vitamin K2 with vitamin D in a paper discussing the vitamins' contributions to reducing the COVID-19 mortality rate. He stated, "Oral supplementation of D3 is the easiest means to prevent deficiencies."

A frequent argument against supplementation of vitamin D3 is that an increased intake could lead to a vitamin D toxicity, also called hypervitaminosis D. This again can cause hypercalcemia, which is the buildup of calcium in the blood leading to vascular calcification, osteoporosis, and kidney stones. However, it has been reported that the reason for hypercalcemia rather lies in a vitamin K2 deficiency, as K2 activates the bone gamma-carboxyglutamic acid-containing protein (osteocalcin) through carboxylation. Activated osteocalcin deposits calcium in the bones, whereas non-activated osteocalcin inhibits calcium absorption by the bones. As the osteocalcin synthesis rate is increased by higher 25(OH)D serum levels, vitamin K2 is required as a natural antagonist."[40]

---

40. Goddek, Simon. "Vitamin D3 and K2 and Their Potential Contribution to Reducing the COVID-19 Mortality Rate," *International Journal of*

Building Stronger Immunity Through Better Nutrition

We've discussed how important vitamins D and K2 are to our bodies and immune systems, generally and in relation to COVID-19. We focused mostly on what may happen when you're deficient in these nutrients. So, does that mean most of us have no reason to be concerned?

Not at all. In our modern lives in the Western world, many people tend to think if they eat enough food, they are getting the nutrients they need. Not so—as I discussed in chapter 2, this is far from true. Our modern lives put us under so much stress and expose us to so many environmental toxins that we need more nutrients than ever. Stress in combination with busy schedules often result in poor food choices. In addition, fresh food has fewer nutrients than ever before.

Moreover, when it comes to vitamins D and K2, there are few food sources available to give us the amounts we need through diet alone.

Many of us are not getting the nutrients we need.

The Prevalence of Vitamin D and Vitamin K2 Deficiencies

The deficiency data for vitamins D and K2 is a reason for real concern.

Vitamin D Deficiency Rates

First, what is considered deficiency?

- People are considered to have severe vitamin D deficiency (risk of rickets) with serum 25(OH)D concentrations in the blood of less than 12 ng/mL.

Infectious Diseases, October 1, 2020, 99: 286–90. https://doi.org/10.1016/j.ijid.2020.07.080

- People are considered to have vitamin D deficiency (inadequate levels for bone and overall health) at serum 25(OH)D concentrations between 12 and 20 ng/mL.
- People generally have sufficient levels for bone health at serum 25(OH)D concentrations of 20 ng/mL or above.[41]

A 2020 study on vitamin D deficiency stated that an estimated one billion people worldwide have vitamin D deficiency.

Breaking this down further, the study noted that 35 percent of the general adult population in the U.S. has vitamin D deficiency, and 50-60 percent of nursing home residents and hospitalized patients have deficiency. Deficiency is 35 percent higher in obese subjects irrespective of latitude and age, and also higher in African American and Hispanic populations.[42]

41. "Vitamin D," National Institutes of Health, U.S. Department of Health & Human Services, updated October 9, 2020: https://ods.od.nih.gov/factsheets/VitaminD-HealthProfessional/

42. Sizar, Omeed, Swapnil Khare, Amandeep Goyal, Pankaj Bansal, and Amy Givler. *Vitamin D Deficiency* (Treasure Island, FL: StatPearls Publishing, 2020). https://www.ncbi.nlm.nih.gov/books/NBK532266/

These numbers are fairly stark—to think that 35 percent of the adult population in a wealthy country like the U.S. is deficient in a well-known nutrient. And that isn't taking into account everyone who is at risk of suboptimal levels. (The level that is optimal may be above what is considered nondeficient; this is an ongoing area of investigation.)

Vitamin K2 Deficiency Rates

Deficiency rates of vitamin K2 are not as clearly defined because the vitamin can't reliably be measured directly in the blood. Instead, vitamin K2 sufficiency is measured indirectly by the concentration of activated K-dependent proteins. Testing vitamin K2 levels just isn't common, but the data we do have points to common and widespread deficiency. It's likely that vitamin K2 deficiency is at much higher rates than vitamin D deficiency.

A recent study analyzed 896 blood samples from healthy adult subjects for carboxylated (activated) and uncarboxylated (unactivated) K-dependent proteins. The study results showed that coagulation proteins were completely carboxylated (made active) by vitamin K. However, a high concentration of other Gla proteins (including osteocalcin and matrix Gla protein) were present in their uncarboxylated forms, in the majority of the subjects investigated.

Uncarboxylated osteocalcin (ucOC) and uncarboxylated matrix Gla protein (ucMGP) are functional laboratory parameters (meaning they can be reliably measured) that indicate a vitamin K deficiency when present. These two proteins in their uncarboxylated forms are associated with an increased risk of bone fractures and vascular complications. This study indicated that the majority of the population as represented by the study subjects had an inadequate supply of vitamin K.[43]

The modern Western diet doesn't typically contain many foods that are good sources of K2, so this isn't surprising. (K1 is much more common in dietary sources.)

> **It's likely that many of us, unless we're actively supplementing with K2, have some level of insufficiency.**

Getting Enough of Vitamins D and K2

By now you understand the need for vitamins D and K2 to ensure a strong immune system response, in general and especially relating to COVID-19. More than ever, this is not the time to be deficient in these micronutrients. Yet many people most likely are, as the data around nutritional deficiency in vitamin D and vitamin K2 suggests.

---

43. Theuwissen, E., E.J. Magdeleyns, and L.A. Braam. "Vitamin K Status in Healthy Volunteers," *Food & Function*, February 2014, 5(2): 229–34. https://pubmed.ncbi.nlm.nih.gov/24296867/

I'd also like to underscore the fact that just because you might not have tipped into full-blown deficiency in a nutrient doesn't mean you are fully sufficient. There's significant space in between the two. Unless you supplement these nutrients already or eat an unconventional daily diet, you almost certainly would benefit from intentionally taking in more of these essential micronutrients.

As with most micronutrients, you can get what you need in two ways: through dietary sources and through supplementation. Dietary choices are always my first preference when possible, but in the cases of vitamins D and K2, it can be difficult to take in sufficient levels this way. Still, let's talk about the options.

Dietary Sources of Vitamin D

A few foods are fortified with vitamin D. This might lead you to expect it's easy to get enough of this vitamin through your diet. Yet most fortified foods contain small amounts, in the form of D2 (ergocalciferol), as it's cheaper to produce. This form isn't easily absorbed by the body.

D3 (cholecalciferol) is the form of vitamin D produced through your skin, and it is the form that raises blood levels of vitamin D most effectively.

Good sources of vitamin D3 include:

- Oily fish
- Fish oil

- Liver
- Egg yolks
- Butter

If these are foods you can add into your diet, I recommend doing so.

Dietary Sources of Vitamin K2

As I mentioned, there aren't many foods rich in vitamin K2 that are common in the modern Western diet. However there are a few options to note.

Dietary sources include:

- Natto (a Japanese fermented soybean dish)
- Egg yolks
- High-fat dairy products
- Other fermented foods (although vitamin K2 content can vary based on the bacteria used in fermentation)

Of these, the K2 MK-7 form is present in fermented foods and dairy products.

Amounts of Vitamins K1 and K2 in Various Foods

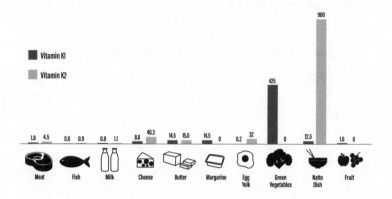

While food sources of vitamin K1 are plentiful, sources for
K2 are more limited or provide only small amounts.

The Value of Supplementation

While I believe we should always take in as many nutrients as
possible through diet, I also know supplementation is a great
way to fill in gaps. This is also Dr. Myers' position.

In his long career centered on nutrition, Dr. Myers has
become passionate about the benefits of supplements. That's
because of what we touched on earlier—our bodies today
need more nutrients than ever, but we're giving them less.
He compares our bodies to vehicles and the food we eat
is the fuel that keeps us going. Modern stresses and toxins
mean that even in periods of little activity, when we should
be idling, we are instead revving the engine to capacity. We
need more gas to do this, yet the gas we're filling up with gets

fewer miles to the gallon than it used to. Think back to the study on fruits and vegetables produced today: they contain up to 40 percent less vitamins and minerals than they did 50 years ago.[44]

Almost all of us need some supplementation.

In the case of vitamins D and K2, supplementation is especially useful.

Our Recommendation: Supplement to Reach Sufficient Levels of Vitamins D and K2

For most vitamins, food sources alone are not only a viable option to meet your nutritional needs, they are preferable. With vitamins D and K2, which we now know are so important to our immune health, the research is showing us that food sources aren't cutting it. Realistically, most of us won't get enough vitamins D and K2 from our diets to be sufficient, allow our immune systems to function at their best, and help us stay healthy through COVID-19 or another pandemic.

Let's look at vitamin K2 as an example. The minimum recommended intake of vitamin K2 is 75 micrograms daily—and this may not even be enough to fully support our

44. Davis, D.R., M.D. Epp, and H.D. Riordan. "Changes in USDA Food Composition Data for 43 Garden Crops, 1950 to 1999," *Journal of the American College of Nutrition*, December 2004, 23(6): 669-82. https://pubmed.ncbi.nlm.nih.gov/15637215/; Davis, D.R. "Declining Fruit and Vegetable Nutrient Composition: What Is the Evidence?" *Hort. Science*, February 2009, 44(1): 15-19. https://journals.ashs.org/hortsci/view/journals/hortsci/44/1/article-p15.xml

immune systems, especially if we have been deficient up to this point. Plus, it's difficult to get that amount in almost any standard Western diet, even a healthy one. To get a sense of why this is, we can look at the vitamin content available in the best food sources.

The only food that easily provides the daily minimum recommended amount of vitamin K2 in a modest serving size is natto, a fermented soybean dish. About 3.5 ounces (100 grams) of natto yields more than the daily minimum of vitamin K2. In the U.S., natto isn't common. It's unlikely to be in our refrigerators or even in our grocery stores. Even if you find it, do you realistically want to eat this food nearly every day? For most of us, the answer is no.

Other foods that are considered some of the best sources of vitamin K2 include egg yolks and certain cheeses. About 3.5 ounces of egg yolks yields 32 micrograms of K2. One egg yolk is around half an ounce, so that means if you eat seven egg yolks in a day, you will have reached half the minimum recommended amount. If you want to round it out with another food that offers any significant amount of vitamin K2, you could eat it with 3.5 ounces of certain cheeses. That is a daily commitment to half a block of cheese and seven egg yolks, just to get the minimum.

The amount of vitamin K2 in other meat and fish is nearly negligible. Green vegetables, which are powerhouses of nutrition generally, offer none. Meat provides some, but to get the daily minimum from meat, you would have to eat almost 60 ounces of it.

This is why so many of us are deficient in vitamin K2.

When you don't have enough of a nutrient in your body, the processes that rely on that nutrient can't function well. The processes that rely on vitamin K2, as well as vitamin D, are so closely tied to your immune system that if you are deficient in them, your immune system will not work as it should.

We need to take in nutrients regularly at levels that keep our systems functioning at their peak. Daily supplementation of a few valuable nutrients can be a great way to make this a consistent part of our lives.

Dr. Myers and Dr. McComsey Recommend

Knowing this, here is what Dr. Myers and I recommend. We suggest you add a supplement of vitamin D and vitamin K2 to your daily routine. Remember that these two work as a perfect pair, and it's safer to take vitamin D along with vitamin K2. So don't choose one of them. Maintain that synergy and take both together. Our recommendation for vitamin K2 is higher than the 75-100 mcg per day you may see as the standard daily dose, and in certain cases higher doses of vitamin K2 (up to 200 mcg per day) might be recommended, especially during the COVID-19 pandemic.

In terms of dosage, we recommend taking the following:
- **2,000 to 4,000 IU per day of vitamin D (make sure it's D3)**
- **100 to 200 mcg per day of vitamin K2 (choose an all-trans form of K2 MK-7)**

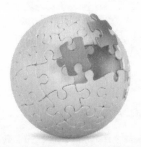

If you already take supplements, this will be a simple addition to your routine. If you don't take anything currently, I suggest connecting it to another part of your daily routine as you build the habit. An easy way to do this is to take it whenever you first head into the kitchen—to make coffee, have breakfast, or get your kids' lunches packed. Post a note for yourself on the cupboard if you have trouble remembering each day.

One important note if you take an anticoagulant drug

Newer generation anticoagulant drugs such as Dabigatran®, Rivaroxaban®, and Apixaban® don't interfere with vitamin K function, but some older anticoagulants can have a dangerous interaction with K. This doesn't necessarily mean you can't take K, but it does mean you should work closely with your doctor or pharmacist to determine how and if it might be safe for you. Please consult your doctor before taking any vitamin K.

The U.S. Pharmacopeial Convention states, "In summary, there is a risk of interaction between MK-7 or other forms of vitamin K and warfarin or other anticoagulant therapy. However, through dose titration and patient counseling, the physician or pharmacist may be able to mitigate that risk to maintain stable anticoagulation control, so long as the patients' vitamin K intake is known."[45]

45. Marles, Robin J., Amy L. Roe, and Hellen A. Oketch-Rabah. "U.S. Pharmacopeial Convention Safety Evaluation of Menaquinone-7, a Form of

Research suggests that being deficient in either or both of these vitamins poses real health risks—especially while in a pandemic. Finding a way to make taking these supplements an ongoing habit that can strengthen your immunity is worth it. While it requires effort, it truly is one of the easiest actions you can take to support your health.

You need to do this before you get sick. Please don't wait for COVID, heart disease, or a bone fracture to start considering these supplements. The best time to do so is now, as part of a well-informed preventative approach.

Vitamin K2 MK-7 Supplement Standards and Purity

If you take vitamin K2 MK-7 as a supplement, you need to find a high-quality version that meets certain essential standards.

Vitamin K2 MK-7 is available in structurally different cis and trans forms, which refers to the structural configuration of the carbon side chain on the molecule. It is essential to choose vitamin K2 in an all-trans form (all-trans MK-7) because the cis form is almost completely ineffective. This is because of the cis form's geometrical alignment: it cannot dock with the relevant enzymes. The enzymes' keys do not fit into the lock of the cis form of vitamin K2. Only the trans form is 100 percent bioactive. For this reason, you'll want to look for a ratio of less than two percent cis with the majority being trans.

Vitamin K," *Nutrition Reviews*, July 1, 2017, 75(7): 553–78. https://pubmed. ncbi.nlm.nih.gov/28838081/

Standards of Supplement Purity

U.S. Pharmacopeia (USP) establishes an independent standard for purity of supplements, and you can be confident that a supplement is pure and of high quality if it has USP on the label. USP sets quality, purity, strength, and identity standards for medicines, food ingredients, and dietary supplements. USP publishes documentary standards (also known as monographs) in their primary reference text, the *USP-NF* (U.S. Pharmacopeia-National Formulary), and by developing USP Reference Standards (also known as physical standards)—used by drug manufacturers to test their products against USP standards to ensure they meet published specifications.

Dr. Myers recommends USP certified supplements as the highest quality and most effective for you to use.

Supplement Purity Standards From the U.S. Pharmacopeia Provide Independent Verification for Vitamin K2 MK-7

Parameter		USP
trans-Menaquinone-7	NLT	96.0%
cis-Menaquinone-7	NMT	2.0%
Menaquinone-6	NMT	2.0%

The U.S. Pharmacopeia has defined the purity of vitamin K2 MK-7 as described. "NLT" = not less than and "NMT" = not more than. The cis form is a biologically inactive contaminant.

Many of the USP standards are enforceable by the United States Food and Drug Administration (FDA) under U.S. law, but USP's independent status means their standards-setting activities are guided only by impartial, empirical, scientific evidence, and public health concerns.

CHAPTER 7

Simple Steps to Power Immune Health

This book was inspired by the emerging research on vitamins D and K2 in regard to COVID-19. These vitamins are powerhouses, and we need more public awareness around them to help support our health now and into the future.

Other Essential Nutrients to Boost Your Health

However, that doesn't mean other micronutrients are not important. We need all of them, and other nutrients can also be important to the immune system. These include the following:

- **Lysine**: An essential amino acid that helps the body absorb calcium, iron, and zinc; promotes collagen growth; helps produce enzymes, antibodies, and hormones; and supports the immune system. Good dietary sources include meat, specifically red meat, pork, and poultry; cheese, particularly hard cheeses; fish; eggs; tofu; and legumes.[46]

---

46. Dresden, Danielle. "What Are the Health Benefits of Lysine?" *Medical News Today*, December 17, 2018: https://www.medicalnewstoday.com/articles/324019#health-benefits

- **Taurine**: An amino acid that plays a role in regulating calcium levels in certain cells, balancing electrolytes in the body, and supporting the development of the nervous system. Good dietary sources include shellfish, especially scallops, mussels, and clams; fish; and dark meat of turkey and chicken.[47]

- **Zinc**: An essential mineral used in immune function, healing wounds, correctly synthesizing DNA, and promoting growth during childhood. (Some early data suggest that zinc supplements may also be important in preventing severe COVID-19. Research here is still ongoing, including at my site in Cleveland.) Good dietary sources include oysters, red meat, poultry, beans, nuts, whole grains, and dairy products.[48] It's important to note that phytates in some dietary sources of zinc—like whole grain breads, cereals, and legumes—bind zinc and inhibit its absorption, making it less bioavailable.

- **Selenium**: A trace mineral that contributes to thyroid hormone metabolism, DNA synthesis, cognitive function, fertility, and the immune system. Good dietary sources include brazil nuts, seafood, and organ meats.[49]

47. Johnson, Jon. "How Does Taurine Affect the Body?" *Medical News Today*, October 17, 2019: https://www.medicalnewstoday.com/articles/326714#taurine-roles-in-the-body

48. Nordqvist, Joseph. "What Are the Health Benefits of Zinc?" *Medical News Today*, updated January 27, 2021: https://www.medicalnewstoday.com/articles/263176#benefits

49. Ware, Megan. "Selenium: What It does and How Much You Need," *Medical News Today*, January 12, 2018: https://www.medicalnewstoday.com/articles/287842

- **Magnesium**: A mineral used to help with muscle and nerve function, regulating blood pressure, and supporting the immune system. Deficiency is common. Adequate amounts of magnesium are required for bone health and work in concert with vitamin D and calcium. Good dietary sources include almonds, spinach, soy milk, black beans, and whole grains.[50]

- **Vitamin A**: A fat-soluble vitamin needed for growth and development, cell recognition, immune function, and reproduction. Good dietary sources include liver, fish oils, leafy green vegetables, orange and yellow vegetables, tomatoes, and fruits.[51]

- **Vitamin C**: A water-soluble vitamin used for wound healing; the immune system; and to help form and maintain bones, skin, and blood vessels. Good dietary sources include citrus fruits, tomatoes, potatoes, red peppers, kiwi, and strawberries.

- **Vitamin E**: A fat-soluble vitamin needed for vision; reproduction; and the health of your blood, brain, and skin. Good dietary sources include plant-based oils, nuts, seeds, fruits, and vegetables.[52]

I suggest you find ways to bring more of these other immunity-supporting micronutrients into your diet, whether

50. Ware, Megan. "Why Do We Need Magnesium?" *Medical News Today*, January 6, 2020: https://www.medicalnewstoday.com/articles/286839#sources

51. Ware, Megan. "Everything You Need to Know about Vitamin A," *Medical News Today*, January 4, 2021: https://www.medicalnewstoday.com/articles/219486

52. "Vitamin E," MayoClinic.org, November 13, 2020: https://www.mayoclinic.org/drugs-supplements-vitamin-e/art-20364144

through dietary sources or daily supplementation. Minerals in particular are at greater risk of being deficient in the diet and they support your immune system as well.

What's the difference between a water-soluble vitamin and a fat-soluble vitamin?

Water-soluble vitamins are readily absorbed into tissues for immediate use. They aren't stored in the body, so they need to be replenished regularly. Any excess is excreted through the urine. Cooking food in water can extract water-soluble vitamins into the cooking water, which may be poured down the sink and lost.

Fat-soluble vitamins are transported by being absorbed by fat globules and carried through the bloodstream. Any excess is stored in the liver or in fatty tissue, so these can sometimes build up to toxic levels. (Vitamin K2 is an exception here, as it holds no risk of overdose.) These vitamins are better absorbed when eaten with fats. For example, vitamin K1, available in salad greens, is better absorbed when a high-fat salad dressing is part of the meal.

Five Daily Habits to Strengthen Your Immune System

We've talked in depth about how essential vitamin D, vitamin K2, and other nutrients are to the body and immune health. We've also touched on a few other aspects of a healthy lifestyle to support immunity. I hope by now you've gotten a sense of how important immune health is. We've been putting this puzzle together piece by piece. Now I'd like to offer further guidance on how to move forward with a holistic approach.

I believe supplementing with vitamins D and K2 is one of the most important things we can do right now, and it needs to be talked about. That's why Dr. Myers and I have written this book. At the same time, I want you to know there's more you can and should do to strengthen your immunity.

Dr. Myers has spent his career in preventative medicine, and one of the greatest observations he's made is that some basic lifestyle choices make a significant difference in our health.

Dr. Myers recommends five simple actions that can establish a strong foundation for better health and immunity, and I find value in including them here. As I first discovered during my clinical rotations with the U.S.-trained infectious disease doctor, the simplest answers are often the best ones.

We suggest you integrate the following habits into your lifestyle, along with ensuring adequate intake of vitamin D and vitamin K2.

1. Drink More Water

After oxygen, water is the most vital nutrient your body needs. Unlike oxygen, your body doesn't just take it in automatically. Yet many people don't even think about drinking water. They'll drink the occasional glass or two, but otherwise, they choose something that satisfies their desire for taste (or caffeine or alcohol) before satisfying their body's need for hydration.

It's true you get some water from most other drinks, as well as from food. In the Western world, you are unlikely to die of dehydration. Yet nothing replaces the original, pure source. Being hydrated enough to survive is not the same as being hydrated enough for your body to function at its best.

Water promotes healthy circulation, clears away toxins, aids digestion, regulates your temperature, and lubricates your joints. What does water have to do with the immune system? Almost every biochemical reaction of almost every cell in your body uses water—and your immune system requires a large number of reactions.

In addition, critical nutrients that supply the immune system are transported through the body in your bloodstream, and that bloodstream is about 90 percent water. You need water to keep things moving. Water also increases blood volume; without enough blood volume, the heart has to work harder, which can cause high blood pressure and inflammation in blood vessels. Inflammation, as we've touched on, is not healthy for the body, and doesn't help your immunity.

Water also supports the lymphatic system, which is an important part of the immune system, and helps the body eliminate toxins that can make you sick. On top of this, drinking juice or soda or almost anything instead of water or herbal tea makes your digestive system work harder as it tries to extract the hydration the body needs. This takes energy that could be going toward a healthy and strong immune response.

Drinking more water is really one of the best things you can do for your body. It may take some effort at first, but once you've made the shift, it becomes almost automatic.

How much water is enough?

You have probably heard that you need eight glasses of water a day. That's a reasonable place to start, especially if your body is on the smaller side. Yet many of us will need more than this.

To get an accurate sense of how much water, in ounces, your body needs per day, just take your body weight in pounds and divide it by two. Divide that by eight to see how many eight-ounce glasses of water you need. (Tall drinking glasses, when filled, are often closer to 10 or 12 ounces, so keep this in mind as you set a water target for yourself.)

When you start drinking this much water, you might have to go to the bathroom more often. That's because your kidneys are used to functioning on the amount of water they've been getting, and when they get more, they need some time to adjust. Give yourself some time to adapt; soon it will balance out, and your body will thrive on the extra hydration.

2. Eat Fresh

We've already spent some time discussing the importance of getting nutrition through diet, but I'd like to go into more detail. It's a critical point. You simply can't eat junk and then expect your body to function well.

As I mentioned earlier in the chapter on nutrition as a foundation for strong immunity, when many of us think about a healthy diet, we think primarily about what we *shouldn't* eat. Or, we just think about getting enough protein, which our bodies do need. While there are plenty of foods (like sugar!) that our bodies do better without, this deeply ingrained mentality is limiting.

This is an essential concept I hope you take away from this book:

For a healthy diet that supports your immunity, you need a steady, adequate supply of micronutrients. It's not all about calories, protein, carbohydrates, and fat—even though that's what you'll hear talked about most often.

For almost everyone, this requires some supplementation, especially where vitamin D and vitamin K2 are concerned, since there are so few food sources of these vitamins that people realistically can eat to obtain them. Even with supplementation, you still need to eat a wide variety of fresh food.

To take in more micronutrients through daily food choices, you need to eat more whole, unprocessed, fresh food, and especially fruits and vegetables. Choose organic when you can.

Five servings of fruits and vegetables has long been used as a daily recommended minimum, and I suggest this be a true minimum. Try to eat closer to 10 servings on most days if you can. This might sound like a lot, but servings can add up more easily than you might expect when you think in terms of what you can add to your diet instead of what you need to replace.

You don't necessarily need to think, "I've got to replace my breakfast with a big bowl of fruit." Or, "I need to have a big salad for lunch instead of the sandwich that's my daily go-to." You can supply your body and immune system with micronutrients just by adding good choices. If you enjoy oatmeal for breakfast and your body responds well to fruit, mix in some berries or apples. Add a green salad to your lunch. Top your pizza with more veggies than usual. If you make regular additions like this second nature, you'll be providing for your body in a new way without having to give anything up. This adding-in approach is subtle, and the results may not be immediately visible. However, the effect is real. It can be transformative for your health.

The more you have these fresh foods on hand, the easier it will be to eat more of them. You may have heard this before, but it's worth repeating: Shop the perimeter of the grocery store. This is where you're generally going to find the least processed, most nutrient-dense foods. Choose a variety of colors so you can eat the rainbow—each color represents different nutrients, so this is an easy way to get a wide variety. Bring these nutrient-rich foods home, and then eat them!

A note on fiber

Another benefit from eating more fresh food is that you'll substantially increase your fiber intake, something the majority of people should do. Kids and adults need between 20 and 30 grams of fiber a day, but most only get about 15 grams.

Fiber helps you feel full faster, it helps regulate blood sugar, and it appears to reduce the risk of several diseases and conditions, including metabolic syndrome, heart disease, and diabetes.[53] Eating enough of it can also help you lose weight.[54] Being overweight puts you at risk for many health conditions, in addition to being a risk factor for more severe COVID-19 outcomes (likely because it is associated with deficiency in vitamins D and K2).

53. "Fiber," *The Nutrition Source*, Harvard T.H. Chan School of Public Health: https://www.hsph.harvard.edu/nutritionsource/carbohydrates/fiber/

54. Ferrari, Nancy. "Making One Change—Getting More Fiber—Can Help with Weight Loss," *Harvard Health Blog*, Harvard Health Publishing, February 17, 2015: https://www.health.harvard.edu/blog/making-one-change-getting-fiber-can-help-weight-loss-201502177721

3. Move Daily

You may think of movement in terms of going running or doing cardio at the gym five times a week, 30 minutes a session. That is great, but physical activity is something our bodies were designed to get throughout the course of a normal day. Granted, what normal days used to look like is a lot different than what they look like today, which is why we tend to be more deliberate about it now and call this need for regular movement "exercise."

It's still possible, though, to incorporate healthy amounts of physical activity into your day by simply moving more: parking farther away from the building, taking a walk around your neighborhood after dinner, gardening, or playing tag with your kids. Add in regular cardio if you can. Make a habit of moving more often throughout your day. Now that more people are at home for large parts of their days, it's even more important to be conscious of this.

Movement or exercise is universally regarded as important to your health, but that doesn't mean we all do it. We're more likely to do something when we really take to heart what's at stake. So even though you already know it's part of a healthy lifestyle, I want to underscore its value here.

When you're deciding if you should take an evening walk around the block or watch an episode of TV instead, consider some of the following benefits. Exercise can:

- Provide short-term benefits to brain health
- Reduce your risk of depression and anxiety

- Help you sleep better (which also has a great effect on your immune system—more on that below)
- Help you maintain your weight and lose weight, if needed
- Lower your cholesterol and improve your blood pressure
- Reduce your risk of developing type 2 diabetes and metabolic syndrome
- Help you control your blood sugar levels
- Lower your risk of developing certain cancers
- Strengthen your bones and muscles
- Decrease inflammation in your body
- Improve your memory and your cognition
- Support your immune system
- Increase your chances of living longer

I'd like to explore those last two points a little further.

How does movement support your immune system? First, it does so by supporting your overall health. This in turn naturally supports your immune health. Second, it may help through encouraging healthy circulation (just like water does).[55]

Third, during regular physical exercise, your body goes through certain changes that encourage a strong immune response: inflammatory responses and stress hormones are decreased, while essential immune cells are at higher levels.

---

55. "Helpful Ways to Strengthen Your Immune System and Fight Off Disease," *How to Boot Your Immune System* (blog), Harvard Health Publishing, updated April 6, 2020: https://www.health.harvard.edu/staying-healthy/how-to-boost-your-immune-system

This leads to improved immunovigilance and a reduction in the systemic inflammation process, both of which can help prevent respiratory diseases, such as (but not limited to) COVID-19.[56]

Exercise also increases your chances of living longer. Take note, because this data is pretty dramatic. Being physically active for around 150 minutes a week is associated with a 33 percent lower risk of all-cause mortality when compared with being physically inactive.[57]

Maybe 150 minutes sounds like a lot. If you can't get there, just do what you can at first, and keep trying to add in more, in whatever increments you can—it doesn't need to all come in chunks of 20 minutes or more.

All-or-nothing thinking doesn't help most of us when it comes to movement (or our diets). What will help instead is the realization that every bit of movement, however small, matters for our general health and our immunity.

---

56. Pelinski da Silveira, Matheus, Kimberly Kamila da Silva Fagundes, Matheus Ribeiro Bizuti, Édina Starck, Renata Calciolari Rossi, and Débora Tavares de Resende e Silva. "Physical Exercise as a Tool to Help the Immune System against COVID-19: An Integrative Review of the Current Literature," *Clinical and Experimental Medicine*, July 29, 2020: 1–14. https://www.ncbi.nlm.nih.gov/pmc/articles/PMC7387807/

57. "Benefits of Physical Activity," Physical Activity, Centers for Disease Control and Prevention, reviewed December 2, 2020: https://www.cdc.gov/physicalactivity/basics/pa-health/index.htm

4. Improve Sleep and Rest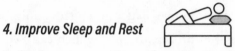

I think most people underestimate the effect sleep has on their body. Of course they know it's healthy, but I don't think they realize what damage can come with not getting enough.

Our culture tends to glorify busyness. Getting by with five or six hours of sleep (or less) and then trying to make up for it with rounds of coffee the next day is almost a status symbol. It's as if it shows how productive or dedicated we are, or how we are prioritizing more important things. However, this is ridiculous because the immune system and your general health critically depend on sufficient sleep.

Sleep is an active process that gives your body a chance to manage its systems, regenerative mechanisms, and immune functions. Many important processes happen while you sleep:

- Your body secretes human growth hormone, which rebuilds muscles
- Your nerve-cell connections strengthen
- Your pulse and breathing rate slow down, which gives your heart and lungs a much-needed chance to rest
- Your digestive system becomes more active, which helps it better absorb nutrients

Even with these functions happening, this period of rest also allows your body to direct more energy into immune function, as it doesn't have to simultaneously support your waking activities. It also improves T-cells in the immune system, which are crucial to fight off infection.

One of my friends often works late nights, and as she's gotten older, she's noticed that almost every time she coasts by on a few hours of sleep, she gets sick the following day. It hasn't been COVID-19 yet, but it's not fun to be sick at all. Especially in today's world, when being sick, whether it's COVID-19 or not, means you need to quarantine until you get a negative COVID-19 test result.

When you don't get the sleep you need, it leads to negative health effects beyond the immune system. It can result in increased weight gain, insulin resistance, cortisol, cardiovascular disease, blood pressure, and inflammation. Getting less than seven hours per night on a regular basis increases stress hormones and adrenaline, essentially leading to a constant or near-constant state of fight-or-flight in the body. Getting less than five hours per night on a regular basis is associated with higher mortality. And when you get less than seven hours of sleep for three nights in a row, the effect is the same as pulling an all-nighter. (This means if you get less than seven hours a night regularly, that's like pulling an all-nighter twice a week, every week. Our bodies are simply not made for that.)

Getting the sleep you need is also necessary for your body to get all it can from your other healthy habits, like eating well and drinking plenty of water.

If at all possible, try to get at least seven hours of sleep every night. Doing this regularly isn't always easy, but as you can see, it's a recommendation I don't make lightly. Sleep matters.

Sleep Cycles

During a sleep cycle, you pass through five stages of brain function.

Stage 1: Your muscle activity begins to slow.

Stage 2: Your eye and muscle movements stop. Your brain waves generally slow.

Stage 3: Your brain activity slows down more. Very slow brain waves called delta waves appear.

Stage 4: Your brain experiences only delta waves. This is considered deep sleep and is harder to wake from.

Stage 5: Brain waves speed up. Here, you experience rapid eye movement (REM) sleep. This is when you dream.

The average adult sleep cycle takes 90-110 minutes.

While the total time slept is essential, as shown by the data here, it's also important you're able to complete full sleep cycles without being awakened in the middle. So, whenever possible, try to create conditions that help you sleep undisturbed.

If you have trouble sleeping through the night, you might want to avoid stimulants like caffeine during the afternoon and evening. Also time any vigorous exercise with sleep in mind: exercising earlier in the day can actually help you fall asleep and sleep better, but try to avoid it within a couple hours of bedtime. Getting enough calcium and magnesium helps encourage healthy sleep, too.

5. Breathe Deeply Every Day

While your breathing is automatic, breathing to your full capacity definitely isn't. Most of us breathe shallowly, in a way that doesn't give your body all the oxygen it could really use, and that then becomes a habit. You can train yourself to breathe differently, to breathe more deeply.

When we breathe deeply, oxygen is provided to brain tissues more fully. The brain requires more oxygen than any other organ, and not getting enough can lead to mental sluggishness, poor mood, and mental health issues. Breathing deeply is also a great way to help manage stress.

This is one of the biggest benefits I'd like to talk about, because Dr. Myers and I both feel passionate about how important it is to find ways to manage stress. In part, that's because when you're experiencing stress, it's not just a state of mind; it's a state of body.

Stress floods your whole body with adrenaline and cortisol to put you in a fight-or-flight state that's designed to help you survive short periods of danger. Your heart rate increases, your breathing quickens, and your blood pressure elevates. It's not a healthy state for your body to stay in long term, yet so many of us live this way. If you experience stress in your life (in other words, if you are a living and breathing human in the modern world), you should learn at least one strategy to help manage it, like conscious, deep breathing.

Long, deep breaths can slow or even stop the stress response by helping you signal to your body the stress has passed and you don't need any more of the adrenaline and cortisol flood. Deep breathing also helps your immunity and serves your body in other ways, such as encouraging clearer thinking, greater creative ability, more restful sleep, faster tissue recovery, and better performance in every body system.

You can and should breathe deeply when you feel particularly overwhelmed by stress, of course, but I recommend also setting aside time to focus on doing this daily. By doing this for just five minutes a day, you help to protect yourself from the negative effects of stress that can build up in your body.

It's really easy to start doing this. Find a quiet place, close your eyes, and start with just five to ten deep breaths in a row. Breathe in deeply through your nose and breathe out deeply through your mouth. Start with the full five minutes if you want, or work up to it. It's that simple.

Fueling Your Immune Power With Five Daily Habits

**Drink
more water**

Eat fresh

Move daily

**Improve sleep
and rest**

**Breathe deeply
every day**

These five daily habits can make a significant difference
in your health over time.

Other Ways to Manage Stress

Deep breathing is one of the easiest things we can do to help manage stress, but there are other excellent methods, too. Some of these include yoga, walking, and mindfulness meditation. In addition to helping manage stress, these activities also provide other health benefits.

Yoga does amazing things for the body. It benefits your heart health and can provide pain relief[58] while also improving flexibility, strength, and balance. It most likely has a beneficial effect on the immune system, too.[59]

Walking is another great activity for managing stress, one that also benefits heart health, supports a healthy weight, and encourages weight loss if needed. It additionally eases joint pain, can curb sugar cravings, and boosts the immune system. One study found that people who walked 20 minutes a day five days a week had 43 percent fewer sick days than people who walked once a week or less. When they did get sick, their symptoms were milder and of shorter duration.[60]

58. "9 Benefits of Yoga," Health, John Hopkins Medicine, accessed January 16, 2021: https://www.hopkinsmedicine.org/health/wellness-and-prevention/9-benefits-of-yoga

59. Gopal, Aravind, Sunita Mondal, Asha Gandhi, Sarika Arora, and Jayashree Bhattacharjee. "Effect of Integrated Yoga Practices on Immune Responses in Examination Stress—A Preliminary Study," *International Journal of Yoga*, January–June 2011, 4(1): 26–32. https://www.ncbi.nlm.nih.gov/pmc/articles/PMC3099098/

60. "5 Surprising Benefits of Walking," *Healthbeat* (blog), Harvard Health Publishing, updated October 13, 2020: https://www.health.harvard.edu/staying-healthy/5-surprising-benefits-of-walking

Mindfulness meditation brings significant benefit as well. Through several well-designed studies, it's been shown to positively impact a few common conditions—including depression, chronic pain, and anxiety.[61] This technique also offers benefit to memory and your ability to concentrate, and it can even help you develop greater compassion and a sense of happiness.[62] A short program of mindfulness has also been shown to have a demonstrable effect on immune function.[63]

Adding one or more of these into your routine along with daily deep breathing will strengthen your immune system even more. These techniques also hold the potential to change your life on levels beyond physical health.

Bringing daily attention to living a healthy lifestyle through these five actions will support your body in amazing ways that complement the nutritional focus of this book. I hope you walk away from this book not just with a deeper understanding of vitamins D and K2, but also with the intention to live in a healthier way overall.

Earlier, I mentioned that all-or-nothing thinking doesn't help when it comes to exercise or diet. I'd like to repeat that.

61. Powell, Alvin. "When Science Meets Mindfulness," *The Harvard Gazette*, April 9, 2018: https://news.harvard.edu/gazette/story/2018/04/harvard-researchers-study-how-mindfulness-may-change-the-brain-in-depressed-patients/

62. Seppälä, Emma. "20 Scientific Reasons to Start Meditating Today," *Psychology Today*, September 11, 2013: https://www.psychologytoday.com/us/blog/feeling-it/201309/20-scientific-reasons-start-meditating-today

63. Powell, Alvin. "When Science Meets Mindfulness," *The Harvard Gazette*, April 9, 2018: https://news.harvard.edu/gazette/story/2018/04/harvard-researchers-study-how-mindfulness-may-change-the-brain-in-depressed-patients/

Dr. Myers and I have offered five simple lifestyle choices you can make, and I hope you make all of them. I also hope you don't think they need to be taken together as a whole to make a difference—every little bit helps. The more you can do, the better, but each of these daily actions is movement in the right direction. Incorporating any changes in the right direction will make a difference for your body and your immunity, especially when paired with the essential vitamins D and K2.

CONCLUSION

Moving Forward With Health and Hope

We've spent time looking at tiny details like proteins, serum levels, and other complicated study data. Admittedly, as a researcher, I love this sort of thing. Part of the reason I love it is because these tiny cells and samples take on a huge importance when we look at a whole body in the scope of real life. They tell us so much when we take the time to understand them and then consider them as part of the bigger picture.

We've looked at many details and layers up close, and now it's time to bring everything together in a way that helps us move forward.

You live inside your one body, and you can't outrun whatever health challenges meet you there.

Right now, living in a time of pandemic, we are facing significant challenges that make our health feel more important and more threatened than ever. All our previous health worries—cancer, type 2 diabetes, heart disease, seasonal colds and flu—are still around, and now we also have COVID-19 as a threat. Some people die from the disease while some recover with long-term consequences, and many more are anxious and afraid. It's a situation we have to take seriously for the sake of our own bodies and our families as well as for the sake of everyone else.

We don't tend to think of it this way, but it's really true that taking care of ourselves is also taking care of public health. Wearing a mask because you know wearing one makes you less likely to spread disease is a way to take care of yourself and others. In the same spirit, we can also contribute to public health by living a healthier lifestyle.

When we nourish our immune systems, we strengthen them. As more of us develop stronger immunity and less susceptibility to infection, there's less spread of disease. When fewer of us get sick with a virus, that limits the virus's opportunities to spread and ultimately, fewer lives are then lost. It also means healthcare systems can function better.

During this pandemic, hospitals around the world have been stretched to (and sometimes much beyond) their limits. Most Americans couldn't have conceived of arriving at a hospital with an urgent problem only to find there isn't room for them to be admitted, yet this has happened. There were simply too many patients in need of care.

Nourishing our immune health should be an essential part of our collective response to COVID-19, along with vaccines, treatments, social distancing, and masks. A big part of your immune health is having healthy levels of vitamin D and vitamin K2 that allow your system to function optimally. These practices will also serve us well going forward. We're unlikely to be able to prevent the next pandemic, but if we as a society begin to enhance our bodies' immune function with readily available nutrients and healthier lifestyles, we could have a real impact on how a future pandemic unfolds.

Immunity is a power that serves both the greater good and ourselves. For most of us, all that's needed to support our immunity is to let our bodies do what they naturally do. The body has an overwhelming desire to achieve balance and thrive. The body's design is incredible.

To provide what our bodies need, we must live a healthier lifestyle. Get plenty of sleep and exercise. Manage stress levels. Eat a nutrient-dense diet with the micronutrients that help us thrive. In the context of COVID-19 and immune health, that means taking in adequate amount of vitamins D and K2, most likely through high-quality supplements.

Together these two vitamins help your immune system downregulate receptors that the virus needs, downregulate the secretion of cytokines that can cause a toxic storm, and activate proteins that help prevent thrombosis and soft tissue calcification. Without adequate levels of both vitamin D and vitamin K2, your immune system can't do this.

COVID-19 has drawn attention to just how many of us have immune systems that aren't functioning near their peak;

it's drawn attention to how nutrient-depleted we are. It's an opportunity, a wake-up call. If we listen and respond by starting to take a more preventative approach, we could pivot our mindsets to better protect us during this pandemic and way beyond it.

With what we've discovered about how vital vitamins D and K2 are to the COVID-19 puzzle, and with what we know of vitamin D's similar effects on other viruses such as influenza, it is reasonable to think this powerful effect the two vitamins have against COVID-19 will extend to other viruses. We don't know that for certain and can't truly know until much more research is done to investigate vitamin K2 and other viral diseases. That research hasn't happened yet.

The world is only beginning to awaken to the full potential of vitamin K2.

When that research is done, though, I believe we'll discover that vitamins D and K2 support the body in just as dramatic a fashion to fight other viruses as we're learning they do in COVID-19.

Prevention is an amazing thing. Yet so many of us are always in treatment mode—and this can be especially true of physicians. We're so focused on fixing problems that we don't put in the time or effort to prevent them from happening in the first place. It's much harder that way.

If we can successfully move toward a focus on prevention, individually and collectively, we will support our health in so many ways.

COVID-19 is scary. But cancer is scary too. So is type 2 diabetes. These chronic conditions kill people every day. One of the most amazing things about my work in HIV has been seeing the field advance over the past two decades. When I first went into HIV research, a diagnosis was a life sentence. Today, patients may have viral loads so low we call them "undetectable." What patients are often dying of now is type 2 diabetes, heart disease, or cancer, not HIV itself.

I find it remarkable that HIV is less of a death sentence than it was. This is why I love my work as a clinician and a researcher. What's hard to accept is the fact that so many people die of adult-onset diabetes or heart disease, diseases that can be avoided with a healthy lifestyle. It is needless and avoidable.

Diseases like type 2 diabetes (or what we could call deficiency states that have tipped into dysfunction) are dangerous all the time, but even more so in the time of COVID-19.

Two of the most important risk factors for severe COVID-19 beyond vitamin D and vitamin K2 deficiency are obesity and diabetes. With these two health conditions, you are predisposed to a worse outcome with COVID-19, and you are probably predisposed to a worse outcome in any pandemic. Moving into a more preventative mindset that emphasizes supplying your body's needs with better nutrition can help you avoid or improve conditions like these. And that might change the course of your life.

I gravitate toward exploring complex diseases, like HIV or like COVID-19, diseases that may have no rapid or immediate cure, or challenge our understanding. Yet within these spaces, it is still simplicity that really speaks to me—finding the simple, logical answers to complex, difficult questions. With this in mind, I pose the following question.

What simple, logical thing can we do right now in this pandemic to help?

The answer is clear and resounding: encourage vitamin D and vitamin K2 sufficiency. In other words, take these vitamins and tell others about them.

There's absolutely no reason to let people keep dying without offering them these pieces of the puzzle, which hold the chance for hope and better health now and into the future.

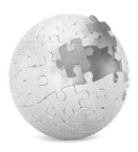

With Appreciation

From Dr. Grace McComsey

To my parents, who made me who I am: My father, who taught me honesty, humility, and integrity, no matter what the situation is—a federal judge who, despite having his life threatened again and again, always took the side of truth. My mother, who decided to put aside work and career to raise me and my three siblings. I do believe this made me a better person. When I was a child, she always made me feel loved and appreciated. As an accomplished professional woman now, I look back on my mother's sacrifice and cherish it even more.

To my husband: You are loving and endlessly supportive. I could not have done it without you!

To my boys: You remind me every day of life's priorities. Thank you.

From Dr. Andrew Myers

For my son and daughter, Drew and Elke.

For Cindy, for all of your love and support.

For Amy Meyer, whose partnership allows me to be professionally passionate every day.

To Robin Bethel and Stacy Ennis for your work as the content team in building out this manuscript for Dr. McComsey and me.

For Maryanna Young and the Aloha Publishing team, Jennifer Regner, Megan Terry, and Heather Goetter, as well as the Fusion Creative Works team, all of whom worked quickly and tirelessly on the production side of this project.

For our publishing attorney, Lloyd Jassin, for your endless support with such a friendly demeanor.

For our publisher, Andy Symonds of Ballast Books, who could see the value of the message and had vision for the project as soon as he heard the results of the studies that informed it.

About the Authors

Dr. Grace McComsey, M.D., FIDSA, is the Vice President of Research and Associate Chief Scientific Officer at University Hospitals (U.H.) Health System in Cleveland, Ohio, a network of 18 hospitals that serves over 1.5 million patients. She is also Professor of Pediatrics and Medicine at Case Western Reserve University.

A board-certified physician with training in adult and pediatric infectious diseases, Dr. McComsey leads the Clinical Research Center at U.H., the central infrastructure for clinical research within the health system. She is also the Chief of the Division of Infectious Diseases at U.H. Rainbow Babies and Children's Hospital.

Dr. McComsey is an internationally known researcher in the field of HIV. She is the author of over 270 peer-reviewed publications in the area of metabolic and cardiovascular complications of HIV infection and its treatment. Dr. McComsey has served as principal investigator on more than 15 grants from the National Institute of Health (NIH), in addition to several foundation and industry grants. She is currently serving as principal investigator on four NIH grants, focusing on aspects of the heightened inflammation and immune activation and its effect on metabolic and cardiovascular comorbidities in adults and children living with HIV.

Dr. McComsey has received several awards as the result of her research, including a Research Award from the HIV Medical Association of the Infectious Diseases Society of America, recognizing her work in HIV metabolic complications, and the YWCA Women of Professional Excellence Award. In July 2020, she received the prestigious Crain's Women of Note award for her commitment to COVID-19 research and for bringing lifesaving treatments to the Cleveland area. Dr. McComsey has earned recognition by her peers and has been regularly voted among the Best Doctors in America and Best Doctors in Cleveland. Additionally she has repeatedly been named one of America's Top Physicians, Top 1 Percent in Healthcare, and among the Exceptional Women in Medicine.

Dr. Andrew Myers is a naturopathic physician with a unique ability to take complex health issues and simplify them, bringing about an understanding that health and wellness are attainable for every individual. He is passionate about creating solutions to the world's prominent health problems by combining the artfulness of natural medicine with the science of the human body.

Dr. Myers has been in private medical practice since 1993. He is a graduate of Bastyr University and completed his residency at the Bastyr Center for Natural Health.

Speaking to audiences worldwide, Dr. Myers communicates the value of taking simple health measures to promote wellness. His genuine manner inspires his listeners to take valuable health-related information and apply it to their daily lives.

As a recognized authority on natural medicines, Dr. Myers is viewed as one of the world's top experts in the formulation of dietary supplements and their scientific substantiation. Dr. Myers formulates complete nutritional lines for global companies and has developed many successful products. He has authored patents ranging from arthritis and weight management to cardiovascular care and pet nutrition.

Acting as coordinator for several clinical trials, Dr. Myers evaluated the effectiveness of natural products in the treatment of obesity, prostate disease, and cardiovascular concerns.

APPENDIX

Additional Studies

Vitamin D

Abdollahi, Alireza, Hasti Kamali Sarvestani, Zahra Rafat, Sara Ghaderkhani, Maedeh Mahmoudi-Aliabadi, Bita Jafarzadeh, and Vahid Mehrtash. "The Association between the Level of Serum 25(OH) Vitamin D, Obesity, and Underlying Diseases with the Risk of Developing COVID-19 Infection: A Case-Control Study of Hospitalized Patients in Tehran, Iran," *Journal of Medical Virology*, 2020: 1-6. https://doi.org/10.1002/jmv.26726

Abrishami, Alireza, Nooshin Dalili, Peyman Mohammadi Torbati, Reyhaneh Asgari, Mehran Arab-Ahmadi, Behdad Behnam, and Morteza Sanei-Taheri. "Possible Association of Vitamin D Status with Lung Involvement and Outcome in Patients with COVID-19: A Retrospective

Study," *European Journal of Nutrition*, October 30, 2020: https://doi.org/10.1007/s00394-020-02411-0

Afshar, Parviz, Mohammad Ghaffaripour, and Hamid Sajjadi. "Suggested Role of Vitamin D Supplementation in COVID-19 Severity," *Journal of Contemporary Medical Sciences*, July-August 2020, 6(4): http://www.jocms.org/index.php/jcms/article/view/822

Alguwaihes, Abdullah M., Mohammed E. Al-Sofiani, Maram Megdad, Sakhar S. Albader, Mohammad H. Alsari, Ali Alelayan, Saad H. Alzahrani, Shaun Sabico, Nasser M. Al-Daghri, and Anwar A. Jammah. "Diabetes and COVID-19 among Hospitalized Patients in Saudi Arabia: A Single-Centre Retrospective Study," *Cardiovascular Diabetology*, December 5, 2020, 19(205): https://doi.org/10.1186/s12933-020-01184-4

Annweiler, Cédric, Bérangère Hanotted, Claire Grandin de l'Epreviere, Jean-MarcSabatier, Ludovic Lafaie, and Thomas Célarier. "Vitamin D and Survival in COVID-19 Patients: A Quasi-Experimental Study," *The Journal of Steroid Biochemistry and Molecular Biology*, November 2020, 204: 105771. https://doi.org/10.1016/j.jsbmb.2020.105771

Annweiler, Gaëlle, Mathieu Corvaisier, Jennifer Gautier, Vincent Dubée, Erick Legrand Guillaume Sacco, and Cédric Annweiler on behalf of the GERIA-COVID study group. "Vitamin D Supplementation Associated to Better Survival in Hospitalized Frail Elderly COVID-19 Patients: The GERIA-COVID Quasi-Experimental Study," *Nutrients*, 2020, 12(11): 3377. https://doi.org/10.3390/nu12113377

Baktash, Vadir, Tom Hosack, Nishil Patel, Shital Shah, Pirabakaran Kandiah, Koenraad Van den Abbeele, Amit K.J. Mandal, and Constantinos G. Missouris. "Vitamin D Status and Outcomes for Hospitalized Older Patients with COVID-19," *Postgraduate Medical Journal* Published Online First, August 27, 2020: https://pmj.bmj.com/content/early/2021/01/23/postgradmedj-2020-138712

Basha, Shaik Lahoor, Sake Suresh, M.D., V.V. Ashok Reddy, M.D., S.P. Surya Teja, Ph.D. "Is the Shielding Effect of Cholecalciferol in SARS-CoV-2 Infection Dependable? An Evidence Based Unravelling," *Clinical Epidemiology and Global Health*, January-March 2021, 9: 326-331. https://www.sciencedirect.com/science/article/pii/S2213398420302256

Benskin, Linda L. "A Basic Review of the Preliminary Evidence That COVID-19 Risk and Severity Is Increased in Vitamin D Deficiency," *Frontiers in Publish Health*, September 10, 2020, 8: 513. https://www.frontiersin.org/articles/10.3389/fpubh.2020.00513/full

Cannell, J.J., R. Vieth, J.C. Umhau, M.F. Holick, W.B. Grant, S. Madronich, C.F. Garland, and E. Giovannucci. "Epidemic Influenza and Vitamin D," *Epidemiol. Infect.*, December 2006, 134(6): 1129-40. doi: 10.1017/S0950268806007175. https://pubmed.ncbi.nlm.nih.gov/16959053/

Carpagnano, G.E., V. Di Lecce, V.N. Quaranta, A. Zito, E. Buonamico, E. Capozza, A. Palumbo, G. Di Gioia, V.N. Valerio, and O. Resta. "Vitamin D Deficiency as a Predictor of Poor Prognosis in Patients with Acute Respiratory Failure Due to COVID-19," *Journal of Endocrinological Investigation*, 2020: https://doi.org/10.1007/s40618-020-01370-x

Castillo, Marta Entrenas, Luis Manuel Entrenas Costa, José Manuel Vaquero Barriosa, Juan Francisco Alcalá Díaz, José López Miranda, Roger Bouillon, and José Manuel Quesada Gomez. "Effect of Calcifediol Treatment and Best Available Therapy versus Best Available Therapy on Intensive Care Unit Admission and Mortality among Patients Hospitalized for COVID-19: A Pilot Randomized Clinical Study," *The Journal of Steroid Biochemistry and Molecular Biology*, October 2020, 203: 105751. https://doi.org/10.1016/j.jsbmb.2020.105751

D'Avolio, Antonio, Valeria Avataneo, Alessandra Manca, Jessica Cusato, Amedeo De Nicolò, Renzo Lucchini, Franco Keller, and Marco Cantù. "25-Hydroxyvitamin D Concentrations Are Lower in Patients with Positive PCR for SARS-CoV-2," *Nutrients*, 2020, 12(5): 1359. https://doi.org/10.3390/nu12051359

De Smet, M.D., Dieter, Kristof De Smet, M.D., Pauline Herroelen, M.Sc., Stefaan Gryspeerdt, M.D., and Geert A. Martens, M.D., Ph.D. "Serum 25(OH)D Level on Hospital Admission Associated with COVID-19 Stage and Mortality," *American Journal of Clinical Pathology*, March 2021, 155(3): 381–388. https://doi.org/10.1093/ajcp/aqaa252

Espitia-Hernandez, Guadalupe, Levy Munguia, Dylan Diaz-Chiguer, Ramiro Lopez-Elizalde, and Fiacro Jimenez-Ponce. "Effects of Ivermectin-Azithromycin-Cholecalciferol Combined Therapy on COVID-19 Infected Patients: A Proof of Concept Study," *Biomedical*

Research, 2020, 31(5). https://www.biomedres.info/
biomedical-research/effects-of-ivermectinazithromycin
cholecalciferol-combined-therapy-on-covid19-infected-
patients-a-proof-of-concept-study-14435.html#corr

Faniyi, Aduragbemi A., Sebastian T. Lugg, Sian E. Faustini,
Craig Webster, Joanne E. Duffy, Martin Hewison, Adrian
Shields, Peter Nightingale, Alex G. Richter, and David
R. Thickett. "Vitamin D Status and Seroconversion for
COVID-19 in UK Healthcare Workers Who Isolated for
COVID-19 Like Symptoms during the 2020 Pandemic,"
medRxiv (Preprint), October 6, 2020: https://doi.
org/10.1101/2020.10.05.20206706

Faul, J.L., C.P. Kerley, B. Love, E. O'Neill, C. Cody, W. Tormey,
K. Hutchinson, L.C. Cormican, and C.M. Burke. "Vitamin
D Deficiency and ARDS after SARS-CoV-2 Infection,"
Irish Medical Journal, 2020, 113(4): 58. http://imj.ie/
vitamin-d-deficiency-and-ards-after-sars-cov-2-infection/

Grant, William B., Henry Lahore, Sharon L. McDonnell,
Carole A. Baggerly, Christine B. French, Jennifer L.
Aliano, and Harjit P. Bhattoa. "Evidence that Vitamin
D Supplementation Could Reduce Risk of Influenza and
COVID-19 Infections and Deaths," *Nutrients*, 2020,
12(4): 988. https://doi.org/10.3390/nu12040988

Hastie, Claire E., Daniel F. Mackay, Frederick Ho, Carlos A. Celis-Morales, Srinivasa Vittal Katikireddia, Claire L. Niedzwiedza, Bhautesh D. Jania, Paul Welsh, Frances S. Maira, Stuart R. Gray, Catherine A. O'Donnell, Jason M.R. Gill, Naveed Sattar, and Jill P. Pell. "Vitamin D Concentrations and COVID-19 Infection in UK Biobank," *Diabetes & Metabolic Syndrome: Clinical Research & Reviews*, July–August 2020, 14(4): 561-565. https://doi.org/10.1016/j.dsx.2020.04.050

Hernández, José L., et al. "Vitamin D Status in Hospitalized Patients with SARS-CoV-2 Infection," *The Journal of Clinical Endocrinology & Metabolism*, October 27, 2020: dgaa733. https://doi.org/10.1210/clinem/dgaa733

Israel, Ariel, Assi Cicurel, Ilan Feldhamer, Yosef Dror, Shmuel M. Giveon, David Gillis, David Strich, and Gil Lavie. "The Link between Vitamin D Deficiency and COVID-19 in a Large Population," *medRxiv* (Preprint), September 7, 2020: https://doi.org/10.1101/2020.09.0 4.20188268

Jain, Anshul, Rachna Chaurasia, Narendra Singh Sengar, Mayank Singh, Sachin Mahor, and Sumit Narain "Analysis of Vitamin D Level among Asymptomatic and Critically Ill COVID-19 Patients and Its Correlation with Inflammatory Markers," *Scientific Reports*, 2020, 10: 20191. https://doi.org/10.1038/s41598-020-77093-z

Jolliffe, David A., et al. "Vitamin D Supplementation to Prevent Acute Respiratory Infections: Systematic Review and Meta-Analysis of Aggregate Data from Randomised Controlled Trials," *medRxiv* (Preprint), November 25, 2020: https://doi.org/10.1101/2020.07.14.20152728

Jungreis, Irwin, and Manolis Kellis. "Mathematical Analysis of Córdoba Calcifediol Trial Suggests Strong Role for Vitamin D in Reducing ICU Admissions of Hospitalized COVID-19 Patients," *medRxiv* (Preprint), December 21, 2020: https://doi.org/10.1101/2020.11.08.20222638

Katz, DMD, Joseph, Sijia Yue, M.Sc., and Wei Xue, Ph.D. "Increased Risk for COVID-19 in Patients with Vitamin D Deficiency," *Nutrition*, April 2021, 84: 111106. https://doi.org/10.1016/j.nut.2020.111106

Kaufman, Harvey W., Justin K. Niles, Martin H. Kroll, Caixia Bi, and Michael F. Holick. "SARS-CoV-2 positivity rates associated with circulating 25-hydroxyvitamin D levels," *PLoS One*, September 1, 2020: https://journals.plos.org/plosone/article?id=10.1371/journal.pone.0239252

Lansiaux, Édouard, Philippe P. Pébaÿ, Jean-Laurent Picard, and Joachim Forget. "COVID-19 and Vit-D: Disease Mortality Negatively Correlates with Sunlight Exposure," *Spatial and Spatio-Temporal Epidemiology*, November 2020, 35: 100362. https://doi.org/10.1016/j.sste.2020.100362

Lau, Frank H., Rinku Majumder, Radbeh Torabi, Fouad Saeg, Ryan Hoffman, Jeffrey D. Cirillo, and Patrick Greiffenstein. "Vitamin D Insufficiency Is Prevalent in Severe COVID-19," *medRxiv* (Preprint), April 28, 2020: https://doi.org/10.1101/2020.04.24.20075838

Ling, Stephanie F., Eleanor Broad, Rebecca Murphy, Joseph M. Pappachan, Satveer Pardesi-Newton, Marie-France Kong, and Edward B. Jude. "High-Dose Cholecalciferol Booster Therapy is Associated with a Reduced Risk of Mortality in Patients with COVID-19: A Cross-Sectional Multi-Centre Observational Study," *Nutrients*, December 11, 2020, 12(12): 3799. https://pubmed.ncbi.nlm.nih.gov/33322317/

Louca, Panayiotis, et al. "Dietary Supplements during the COVID-19 Pandemic: Insights from 1.4M Users of the COVID Symptom Study App—A Longitudinal App-Based Community Survey," *medRxiv* (Preprint),

November 27, 2020: https://doi.org/10.1101/2020.11. 27.20239087

Luo, Xia, Qing Liao, Ying Shen, Huijun Li, and Liming Cheng. "Vitamin D Deficiency Is Associated with COVID-19 Incidence and Disease Severity in Chinese People," *The Journal of Nutrition*, January 2021, 151(1): 98–103. https://doi.org/10.1093/jn/nxaa332

Marik, Paul E., Pierre Kory, and Joseph Varon. "Does Vitamin D Status Impact Mortality from SARS-CoV-2 Infection?" *Medicine in Drug Discovery*, 2020, 6: 100041. https://pubmed.ncbi.nlm.nih.gov/32352080/

Meltzer, M.D., Ph.D., David O., Thomas J. Best, Ph.D., Hui Zhang, Ph.D., Tamara Vokes, M.D., Vineet Arora, M.D., MPP, and Julian Solway, M.D. "Association of Vitamin D Status and Other Clinical Characteristics with COVID-19 Test Results," *JAMA Netw Open*, 2020, 3(9): e2019722. https://jamanetwork.com/journals/ jamanetworkopen/fullarticle/2770157

Mercola, Joseph, William B. Grant, and Carol L. Wagner. "Evidence Regarding Vitamin D and Risk of COVID-19 and Its Severity," *Nutrients*, 2020, 12(11): 3361. https:// www.mdpi.com/2072-6643/12/11/3361

Merzon, Eugene, Dmitry Tworowski, Alessandro Gorohovski, Shlomo Vinker, Avivit Golan Cohen, Ilan Green, and Milana Frenkel-Morgenstern. "Low Plasma 25(OH) Vitamin D Level Is Associated with Increased Risk of COVID-19 Infection: An Israeli Population-Based Study," *The FEBS Journal*, September 2020, 287(17): 3693-3702. https://doi.org/10.1111/febs.15495

Mitchell, M.D., Deborah M., Maria P. Henao, B.A., Joel S. Finkelstein, M.D., and Sherri-Ann M. Burnett-Bowie, M.D., MPH. "Prevalence and Predictors of Vitamin D Deficiency in Healthy Adults," *Endocr. Pract.*, November-December 2012, 18(6): 914–923. https://doi.org/10.4158/EP12072.OR

Mok, Chee Keng, et al. "Calcitriol, the Active Form of Vitamin D, Is a Promising Candidate for COVID-19 Prophylaxis," *medRxiv* (Preprint), June 22, 2020: https://doi.org/10.1101/2020.06.21.162396

Murai, Igor H., et al. "Effect of Vitamin D3 Supplementation vs Placebo on Hospital Length of Stay in Patients with Severe COVID-19: A Multicenter, Double-blind, Randomized Controlled Trial," *medRxiv* (Preprint), November 17, 2020: https://doi.org/10.1101/2020.11.16.20232397

Ohaegbulam, M.D., Ph.D., Kim C., Mohamed Swalih, D.O., Pranavkumar Patel, MBBS, Miriam A. Smith, M.D., FACP, MBA, and Richard Perrin, M.D. "Vitamin D Supplementation in COVID-19 Patients: A Clinical Case Series," *American Journal of Therapeutics*, September/October 2020, 27(5): e485-e490. https://journals. lww.com/americantherapeutics/Abstract/2020/10000/ Vitamin_D_Supplementation_in_COVID_19_Patients __A.8.aspx

Palacios, Cristina, and Lilliana Gonzalez. "Is Vitamin D Deficiency a Major Global Public Health Problem?" *The Journal of Steroid Biochemistry and Molecular Biology,* October 2014, 144, Part A: 138-145. https://www. ncbi.nlm.nih.gov/pmc/articles/PMC4018438/pdf/ni-hms541186.pdf

Panagiotou, Grigorios, Su Ann Tee, Yasir Ihsan, Waseem Athar, Gabriella Marchitelli, Donna Kelly, Christopher S. Boot, Nadia Stock, James Macfarlane, Adrian R. Martineau, Graham Burns, and Richard Quinton. "Low Serum 25-Hydroxyvitamin D (25[OH]D) Levels in Patients Hospitalised with COVID-19 Are Associated with Greater Disease Severity: Results of a Local Audit of Practice," *medRxiv* (Preprint), June 25, 2020: https://doi. org/10.1101/2020.06.21.20136903

Radujkovic, Aleksandar, Theresa Hippchen, Shilpa Tiwari-Heckler, Saida Dreher, Monica Boxberger, and Uta Merle. "Vitamin D Deficiency and Outcome of COVID-19 Patients," *Nutrients* 2020, *12*(9): 2757. https://doi.org/10.3390/nu12092757

Rastogi, Ashu, Anil Bhansali, Niranjan Khare, Vikas Suri, Narayana Yaddanapudi, Naresh Sachdeva, G.D. Puri, and Pankaj Malhotra. "Short Term, High-Dose Vitamin D Supplementation for COVID-19 Disease: A Randomised, Placebo-Controlled, Study (SHADE Study)," *Postgraduate Medical Journal*, published online first November 12, 2020: https://pmj.bmj.com/content/early/2020/11/12/postgradmedj-2020-139065.info

Tan, Chuen Wen, et al. "Cohort Study to Evaluate the Effect of Vitamin D, Magnesium, and Vitamin B12 in Combination on Progression to Severe Outcomes in Older Patients with Coronavirus (COVID-19)," *Nutrition*, November–December 2020, 79-80: 111017. https://doi.org/10.1016/j.nut.2020.111017

Urashima, Mitsuyoshi, Takaaki Segawa, Minoru Okazaki, Mana Kurihara, Yasuyuki Wada, and Hiroyuki Ida. "Randomized Trial of Vitamin D Supplementation to Prevent Seasonal Influenza A in Schoolchildren," *The*

American Journal of Clinical Nutrition, May 2010, 91(5): 1255–1260. https://doi.org/10.3945/ajcn.2009.29094

Van Ballegooijen, Adriana J., Stefan Pilz, Andreas Tomaschitz, Martin R. Grübler, and Nicolas Verheyen. "The Synergistic Interplay between Vitamins D and K for Bone and Cardiovascular Health: A Narrative Review," *International Journal of Endocrinology*, 2017, Article ID 7454376. https://doi.org/10.1155/2017/7454376

Vassiliou, Alice G., Edison Jahaj, Maria Pratikaki, Stylianos E. Orfanos, Ioanna Dimopoulou, and Anastasia Kotanidou. "Low 25-Hydroxyvitamin D Levels on Admission to the Intensive Care Unit May Predispose COVID-19 Pneumonia Patients to a Higher 28-Day Mortality Risk: A Pilot Study on a Greek ICU Cohort," *Nutrients*, December 3, 2020, 12(12): 3773. https://www.mdpi.com/2072-6643/12/12/3773

Walk, Jona, Anton S.M. Dofferhoff, Jody M.W. van den Ouweland, Henny van Daal, and Rob Janssen. "Vitamin D—Contrary to Vitamin K—Does Not Associate with Clinical Outcome in Hospitalized COVID-19 Patients," *medRxiv* (Preprint), November 9, 2020: https://doi.org/10.1101/2020.11.07.20227512

Walrand, Stephan. "The Autumn COVID-19 Surge Dates in Europe Are Linked to Latitudes and Not to Temperature, nor to Humidity, Pointing Vitamin D as a Contributing Factor," *medRxiv* (Preprint), December 2, 2020: https://doi.org/10.1101/2020.10.28.20221176

Ye, Kun, Fen Tang, Xin Liao, Benjamin A. Shaw, Meiqiu Deng, Guangyi Huang, Zhiqiang Qin, Xiaomei Peng, Hewei Xiao, Chunxia Chen, Xiaochun Liu, Leping Ning, Bangqin Wang, Ningning Tang, Min Li, and Fan Xu. "Does Serum Vitamin D Level Affect COVID-19 Infection and Its Severity?—A Case-Control Study," *Journal of American College of Nutrition*, October 13, 2020: 10.1080/07315724.2020.1826005

Vitamin K

Anastasi, Emanuela, Cristiano Ialongo, Raffaella Labriola, Giampiero Ferraguti, Marco Lucarelli, and Antonio Angeloni. "Vitamin K deficiency and COVID-19," *Scandinavian Journal of Clinical and Laboratory Investigation*, 2020, 80: 1-3. 10.1080/00365513.2020.1805122. https://doi.org/10.1080/00365513.2020.1805122

Berenjian, Aydin, Raja Mahanama, John Kavanagh, and Fariba Dehghani. "Vitamin K series: current status and future prospects," *Critical Reviews in Biotechnology*, 2015, 35(2): 199-208. https://doi.org/10.3109/07388551.2013.832142

Berenjian, Aydin, and Zahra Sarabadani. "How Menaquinone-7 Deficiency Influences Mortality and Morbidity among COVID-19 Patients," *Biocatalysis and Agricultural Biotechnology*, 2020, 29: 101792. doi:10.1016/j.bcab. 2020.101792. https://doi.org/10.1016/j.bcab.2020.101792

Castoldi, Elisabetta, and Tilman M. Hackeng. "Regulation of coagulation by protein S," Current Opinion in Hematology, September 2008, 15(5): 529-536. doi: 10.1097/MOH. 0b013e328309ec97. https://journals.lww.com/co-hematol ogy/Abstract/2008/09000/Regulation_of_coagulation_ by_protein_S.15.aspx

Chen, Yunzi, Jing Zhang, Xin Ge, Jie Du, Dilip K. Deb, and Yan Chun Li. "Vitamin D Receptor Inhibits Nuclear Factor kB Activation by Interacting with IkB Kinase β Protein," 2013, *J. Biol. Chem.*, 288(27): 19450-19458. https://www.ncbi.nlm.nih.gov/pmc/articles/PMC370 7648/

Dahlbäck, Björn. "Vitamin K-Dependent Protein S: Beyond the Protein C Pathway," *Semin. Thromb. Hemost.*, March

2018, 44(2): 176-184. doi: 10.1055/s-0037-1604092. https://pubmed.ncbi.nlm.nih.gov/28905350/

De Brouwer, Bart, Michiel Spanbroek, Nadja Drummen, Jody Van Den Ouweland, Pieter Zanen, Cees Vermeer, and Rob Janssen. "Low Vitamin K Status Is Associated with COPD and Accelerated Degradation of Mature Elastin," American Thoracic Society 2016 International Conference Abstracts/B61. Fibroblasts and Matrix in COPD. https://www.atsjournals.org/doi/abs/10.1164/ajrccm-conference.2016.193.1_MeetingAbstracts. A4134

Janssen, Rob, and Jona Walk. "Vitamin K Epoxide Reductase Complex Subunit 1 (VKORC1) Gene Polymorphism as Determinant of Differences in COVID-19-Related Disease Severity," Medical Hypotheses, August 2020, 144: DOI: 10.1016/j.mehy.2020.110218. https://www.researchgate.net/publication/343862973_Vitamin_K_epoxide_reductase_complex_subunit_1_VKORC1_gene_polymorphism_as_determinant_of_differences_in_Covid-19-related_disease_severity

Janssen, Rob, Margot P.J. Visser, Anton S.M. Dofferhoff, Cees Vermeer, Wim Janssens, and Jona Walk. "Vitamin K Metabolism as the Potential Missing Link between

Lung Damage and Thromboembolism in Coronavirus Disease 2019," *British Journal of Nutrition,* 2020: 1-8. doi:10.1017/S0007114520003979. https://pubmed. ncbi.nlm.nih.gov/33023681/

Lal, Neha, and Aydin Berenjian. "Cis and Trans Isomers of the Vitamin Menaquinone-7: Which One Is Biologically Significant?", *Appl. Microbiol. Biotechnol.,* April 2020, 104(7): k2765-2776. doi: 10.1007/s00253-020-10409-1. https://pubmed.ncbi.nlm.nih.gov/32009201/

Linneberg, A., F.B. Kampmann, S.B. Israelsen, L.R. Andersen, H.L. Jørgensen, H. Sandholt, N.R. Jørgensen, S.M. Thysen, and T. Benfield. "Low Vitamin K Status Predicts Mortality in a Cohort of 138 Hospitalized Patients with COVID-19," *medRxiv* (Preprint), December 23, 2020: https://doi.org/10.1101/2020.12.21.20248613

Majid, Zainab, Faryal Tahir, Jawad Ahmed, Taha Bin Arif, and Anwarul Haq. "Protein C Deficiency as a Risk Factor for Stroke in Young Adults: A Review," *Cureus,* March 2020, 12(3): e7472. doi: 10.7759/cureus.7472. https:// www.ncbi.nlm.nih.gov/pmc/articles/PMC7188017/

Padda, Inderbir S., Poras Patel, and Divyaswathi Citla Sridhar. "Protein S and C," [Updated 2020 May 15].

In: *StatPearls* [Internet]. Treasure Island (FL): StatPearls Publishing; 2021 Jan. Available from: https://www.ncbi.nlm.nih.gov/books/NBK557814/

Pan, Min-Hsiung, Katarzyna Maresz, Pei-Sheng Lee, Jia-Ching Wu, Chi-Tang Ho, Janusz Popko, Dilip S. Mehta, Sidney J. Stohs, and Vladimir Badmaev. "Inhibition of TNF-α, IL-1α, and IL-1β by Pretreatment of Human Monocyte-Derived Macrophages with Menaquinone-7 and Cell Activation with TLR Agonists In Vitro," *J. Med. Food.*, 2016, 19(7): 663-669. https://pubmed.ncbi.nlm.nih.gov/27200471/

Reddi, K., B. Henderson, S. Meghji, M. Wilson, S. Poole, C. Hopper, M. Harris, and S.J. Hodges. "Interleukin 6 production by lipopolysaccharide-stimulated human fibroblasts is potently inhibited by naphthoquinone (vitamin K) compounds," *Cytokine*, April 1995, 7(3): 287-90. doi: 10.1006/cyto.1995.0034. https://pubmed.ncbi.nlm.nih.gov/7640347/

Reider, Carroll A., Ray-Yuan Chung, Prasad P. Devarshi, Ryan W. Grant, and Susan Hazels Mitmesser. "Inadequacy of Immune Health Nutrients: Intakes in U.S. Adults, the 2015-2016 NHANES," *Nutrients*, June 2020, 12(6): 1735. https://www.ncbi.nlm.nih.gov/pmc/articles/PMC7352522/

Schurgers, L.J., J.M. Geleijnse, D.E. Grobbee, H.A.P. Pols, A. Hofman, J.C.M. Witteman, and C. Vermeer. "Nutritional Intake of Vitamins K1 (Phylloquinone) and K2 (Menaquinone) in The Netherlands," *Journal of Nutritional & Environmental Medicine*, 1999, 9(2): 115-122. DOI: 10.1080/13590849961717. https://doi.org/10.1080/13590849961717

Schurgers, Leon J., Kirsten J.F. Teunissen, Karly Hamulyák, Marjo H.J. Knapen, Hogne Vik, and Cees Vermeer. "Vitamin K-Containing Dietary Supplements: Comparison of Synthetic Vitamin K1 and Natto-Derived Menaquinone-7," *Blood*, April 15, 2007, 109(8): 3279-83. doi: 10.1182/blood-2006-08-040709. https://pubmed.ncbi.nlm.nih.gov/17158229/

Suleiman, Lutfi, Claude Négrier, and Habib Boukerche. "Protein S: A multifunctional anticoagulant vitamin K-dependent protein at the crossroads of coagulation, inflammation, angiogenesis, and cancer," *Critical Reviews in Oncology/Hematology*, December 2013, 88(3): 637-654. https://doi.org/10.1016/j.critrevonc.2013.07.004. https://www.sciencedirect.com/science/article/abs/pii/S1040842813001558?via%3Dihub

Theuwissen, Elke, Ellen C. Cranenburg, Marjo H. Knapen, Elke J. Magdeleyns, Kirsten J. Teunissen, Leon J.

Schurgers, Egbert Smit, and Cees Vermeer. "Low-Dose Menaquinone-7 Supplementation Improved Extra-Hepatic Vitamin K Status, But Had No Effect on Thrombin Generation in Healthy Subjects," *British Journal of Nutrition*, 2012, 108(9): 1652-1657. doi:10.1017/S0007114511007185. https://www.cambridge.org/core/journals/british-journal-of-nutrition/article/lowdose-menaquinone7-supplementation-improved-extrahepatic-vitamin-k-status-but-had-no-effect-on-thrombin-generation-in-healthy-subjects/D25A8ED353E8F199EEAE9905D716A88E

Van Ballegooijen, Adriana J., Joline W.J. Beulens, Lyanne M. Kieneker, Martin H. de Borst, Ron T. Gansevoort, Ido P. Kema, Leon J. Schurgers, Marc G. Vervloet, and Stephan J.L. Bakker. "Combined Low Vitamin D and K Status Amplifies Mortality Risk: A Prospective Study," *European Journal of Nutrition*, August 17, 2020: https://doi.org/10.1007/s00394-020-02352-8

Walk, Jona, Anton S.M. Dofferhoff, Jody M.W. van den Ouweland, Henny van Daal, and Rob Janssen. "Vitamin D—Contrary to Vitamin K—Does Not Associate with Clinical Outcome in Hospitalized COVID-19 Patients," *medRxiv* (Preprint), November 9, 2020: https://doi.org/10.1101/2020.11.07.20227512

Xia, JingHe, Sachiko Matsuhashi, Hiroshi Hamajima, Shinji Iwane Hirokazu Takahashi, Yuichiro Eguchi, Toshihiko Mizuta, Kazuma Fujimoto, Shun'ichi Kuroda, and Iwata Ozaki. "The role of PKC isoforms in the inhibition of NF-κB activation by vitamin K2 in human hepatocellular carcinoma cells," *The Journal of Nutritional Biochemistry*, December 2012, 23(12): 1668-1675. https://doi.org/10.1016/j.jnutbio.2011.11.010

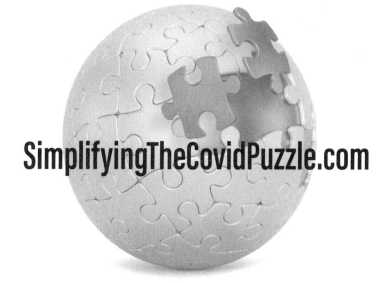

SimplifyingTheCovidPuzzle.com